DEVELOPING NEW CONTRACEPTIVES

Obstacles and Opportunities

Luigi Mastroianni, Jr., Peter J. Donaldson,
and Thomas T. Kane, editors
Committee on Contraceptive Development

Committee on Population
Commission on Behavioral and Social Sciences and Education
National Research Council

and

Division of International Health
Institute of Medicine

NATIONAL ACADEMY PRESS
Washington, D.C. 1990

NATIONAL ACADEMY PRESS • 2101 Constitution Avenue, NW • Washington, DC 20418

NOTICE: The project that is the subject of this report was approved by the Governing Board of the National Research Council, whose members are drawn from the councils of the National Academy of Sciences, the National Academy of Engineering, and the Institute of Medicine. The members of the committee responsible for the report were chosen for their special competences and with regard for appropriate balance.

This report has been reviewed by a group other than the authors according to procedures approved by a Report Review Committee consisting of members of the National Academy of Sciences, the National Academy of Engineering, and the Institute of Medicine.

The National Academy of Sciences is a private, nonprofit, self-perpetuating society of distinguished scholars engaged in scientific and engineering research, dedicated to the furtherance of science and technology and to their use for the general welfare. Upon the authority of the charter granted to it by the Congress in 1863, the Academy has a mandate that requires it to advise the federal government on scientific and technical matters. Dr. Frank Press is president of the National Academy of Sciences.

The National Academy of Engineering was established in 1964, under the charter of the National Academy of Sciences, as a parallel organization of outstanding engineers. It is autonomous in its administration and in the selection of its members, sharing with the National Academy of Sciences the responsibility for advising the federal government. The National Academy of Engineering also sponsors engineering programs aimed at meeting national needs, encourages education and research, and recognizes the superior achievements of engineers. Dr. Robert M. White is president of the National Academy of Engineering.

The Institute of Medicine was established in 1970 by the National Academy of Sciences to enlist distinguished members of the appropriate professions in the examination of policy matters pertaining to the health of the public. The Institute acts under the responsibility given to the National Academy of Sciences by its congressional charter to be an adviser to the federal government and, upon its own initiative, to identify issues of medical care, research, and education. Dr. Samuel O. Thier is president of the Institute of Medicine

The National Research Council was organized by the National Academy of Sciences in 1916 to associate the broad community of science and technology with the Academy's purposes of furthering knowledge and advising the federal government. Functioning in accordance with general policies determined by the Academy, the Council has become the principal operating agency of both the National Academy of Sciences and the National Academy of Engineering in providing services to the government, the public, and the scientific and engineering communities. The Council is administered jointly by both Academies and the Institute of Medicine. Dr. Frank Press and Dr. Robert M. White are chairman and vice chairman, respectively, of the National Research Council.

Library of Congress Cataloging-in-Publication Data

Developing new contraceptives : obstacles and opportunities / Luigi
    Mastroianni, Jr. , Peter J. Donaldson, and Thomas T. Kane, editors ;
    Committee on Contraceptive Development ... [et. al.].
        p.   cm.
    Includes bibliographical references.
    ISBN 0-309-04147-3
    1. Contraceptives—Research—United States. 2. Contraceptive
drugs—Research—United States. I. Mastroianni, Luigi.
II. Donaldson, Peter J. III. Kane, Thomas T., 1951– .
RC137.D48 1990
613.9'4—dc20   89-13654
                                                                                CIP

Copyright © 1990 by the National Academy of Sciences

Printed in the United States of America

Committee on Contraceptive Development

Preface

This report is the work of the Committee on Contraceptive Development, which is jointly staffed and administered by the National Research Council's Committee on Population and the Institute of Medicine's Division of International Health. The report analyzes the process by which contraceptives are developed and approved for use in the United States and suggests ways to change that process to facilitate the development of safer, more effective, more convenient, and more acceptable new contraceptive methods.

The study that produced this report is the most recent manifestation of a commitment by the National Research Council that began nearly 70 years ago with the establishment of its Committee on Research in Problems of Sex, for four decades a major force behind the development of scientific studies of human sexuality. Since then, other Research Council committees and, in this decade, the Institute of Medicine and the National Academy of Engineering have applied continuing analytic attention to a variety of issues related to human reproduction, population growth, and contraception.

This report reviews the effects of factors that are widely believed to have slowed the development of new contraceptives, including the impact of the U.S. tort law system, the federal government's regulatory procedures, the organization of research and development activities, the distribution of scientific personnel and financial resources, as well as attitudes toward the control of reproduction.

The Institute of Medicine and the Committee on Population were asked to undertake this study by the Andrew W. Mellon Foundation. The foundation, which has been a major supporter of reproductive biology and contraceptive development in the United States, had become concerned about the pace at which new products were being brought to the market and asked the committee to review the effects of organizational and policy issues on the contraceptive development process.

The committee that undertook this study was composed of a diverse group of experts who represented a variety of backgrounds, perspectives, and disciplines. As with all committees of the National Research Council and of the Institute of Medicine, care was taken to ensure that the committee was balanced with respect to opinions and expertise related to contraceptive development. Particularly important in this regard was the fact that the scope of the committee's work and membership were reviewed by the Committee on Population as well as by the Commission on Behavioral and Social Sciences and Education and the Institute of Medicine, thus ensuring particularly careful scrutiny at the very earliest stages of the committee's work.

During the course of the study, the Committee on Population reviewed the progress of the committee's work at each of its meetings and took responsibility for reviewing the final report. The Committee on Population also asked outside experts to review portions of the report. In addition, six other experts reviewed the report on behalf of the Commission on Behavioral and Social Sciences and Education and the Institute of Medicine. In short, since its inception, the work of the Committee on Contraceptive Development has been characterized by particularly high standards, broad representation, and careful scrutiny.

In the course of its meetings, the committee heard from representatives of a variety of organizations involved in contraceptive development, including experts from federal government agencies, nonprofit organizations, the university research community, international organizations, and the pharmaceutical industry. The committee learned about contraceptive acceptability and use in the developing world from two of its members, one from sub-Saharan Africa and another from Latin America. The committee also commissioned several background papers on topics related to the development of new contraceptives.

The Institute of Medicine and the Committee on Population appreciate the opportunity provided by the Andrew W. Mellon Foundation to investigate the process of contraceptive development and approval. Mellon Foundation support enabled the Committee on Contraceptive Development to undertake a detailed review of the development process and to carefully examine a variety of potentially important changes to the way contraceptives are developed and regulated. We are very grateful to the members of the Committee on Contraceptive Development, and especially to Luigi Mastroianni, Jr., the committee chair, for their efforts on this report.

ALBERT I. HERMALIN
Chair, Committee on Population

SAMUEL O. THIER
President, Institute of Medicine

Acknowledgments

The committee is particularly grateful to the following people, who presented their views to the committee on the development of new contraceptives: Wayne Bardin of the Population Council, Jose Barzelatto of the World Health Organization, Leon Dash of the *Washington Post*, Gary Gereffi of Duke University, Florence Haseltine of the National Institute of Child Health and Human Development, Gary Hodgen of Eastern Virginia Medical College, Richard Lincoln of the Alan Guttmacher Institute, John McGuire of the Ortho Pharmaceutical Corporation, Malcolm Potts of Family Health International, James Shelton of the Agency for International Development, Solomon Sobel and Bruce Stadel of the Food and Drug Administration, Bruce Vorhauer of Polymed Laboratories, and Koenraad Wiedhaup of Organon International. Their thoughtful presentations and their willingness to provide detailed answers to the committee's questions contributed greatly to the quality of this report. The committee also appreciates the work of Richard Lincoln, Malcolm Potts, and Cynthia Green, who prepared background papers for this report.

The committee especially appreciates the help of specialists who provided data and other information to the committee: Gabriel Bially, Arthur Campbell, Peggy Garner, Florence Hazeltine, Darlene Levenson, George Leverenz, and Ruth Verstieg of the National Institute of Child Health and Human Development; Linda Atkinson and Peter Carpenter of ALZA Corporation; Jacqueline Darroch Forrest, Susan Jew, and Richard Lincoln of the Alan Guttmacher Institute; Henry Gabelnick of the Contraceptive Research and Development program; Laneta Dorflinger and James Shelton of the Agency for International Development; Sheldon Segal of the Rockefeller Foundation; J. Kellum Smith and Carolyn Makinson of the Andrew W. Mellon Foundation; Wayne Bardin, Martha Brady, Oscar Harkavy, and Elsie Millaway of the Population Council; San Balogh, Gary Grubb, Susan McIntyre, Robin Foldesy, and Roberto Rivera of Family Health International; Philip Corfman, Susan Daugherty, Mark Ellengold, Raja Kammala, and Lillian Yin of the Food and Drug Administration; Henry Grabowski of Duke University; Richard Levin of Yale University; Ronald Hansen of the University of Rochester; Steven Wiggins of the University of Texas; John Wundrock and Pat Thome of Wisconsin Pharmacal; Lee Beck and Daniel Lewis of Stolle Research and Development Corporation; Joan Dunlop of the International Women's Health Coalition; Louis Lasagna and Barbara Richard of the Center for Drug Development; Roderick Mackenzie, Mary Kurtz, and Nancy Larson of GynoPharma; Peter Rowe of the World Health Organization; and Jacqueline Sherris and Patti Benson of the Program of Applied Technology in Health.

Staff at the following organizations were also very helpful: Public Citizen; the National Right to Life Committee; the National Human Life Federation; the Kennedy Institute Center for Bioethics; the Pharmaceutical Manufacturers Association; the Food, Drug, and Cosmetic Law Institute; and the Association for Voluntary Surgical Contraception. The products liability attorneys, public relations officers, and directors of research and development and of regulatory affairs at companies involved in contraceptive research or marketing provided whatever information their corporate policies allowed.

We owe particular appreciation to Peter Donaldson, study director, and Thomas Kane, research associate, who helped organize the committee, provided necessary support throughout the study, and assisted with the drafting and coordination of the report. We also thank Anna Boe, who provided a great deal of help with Chapters 7 and 8. We are grateful to Lisa Brecker, who aided the committee by collecting and analyzing data on various aspects of contraceptive development. We also wish to thank Jill Gay, Jennifer Hess, Katherine Kost, Sahr Kpundeh, and Susan Rogers, who assisted the committee in organizing its work. Eugenia Grohman, associate director for reports of the Commission on Behavioral and Social Sciences and Education, critically reviewed the report. Christine McShane, CBASSE editor, edited and significantly improved the report; she also coordinated its review and publication.

This report is truly a committee document. Members of the committee were committed and involved throughout the study, from early drafting through the final revisions. All of my colleagues on the committee made generous contributions of time and expert knowledge; their insights and ideas were pivotal in the development of this report.

LUIGI MASTROIANNI, JR.
Chair, Committee on
Contraceptive Development

Contents

DEVELOPING
NEW
CONTRACEPTIVES

Executive Summary

Currently available contraceptive methods are not well suited to the religious, social, economic, or health circumstances of many Americans and, therefore, a wider array of safe and effective contraceptives is highly desirable. Important individual and social benefits are associated with lower rates of abortion and unwanted pregnancy, especially among teenagers, that new contraceptive methods might help to bring about. The Committee on Contraceptive Development was appointed to explore organizational and policy issues affecting the development of such new contraceptive technologies.

THE NEED FOR NEW CONTRACEPTIVES

The committee found that important changes have taken place in contraceptive research and development over the past two decades. All but one of the large U.S. pharmaceutical companies formerly conducting research on new contraceptives have withdrawn from the field. Partly as a result of this change, and partly as a consequence of changing patterns of support from the federal government, nonprofit organizations and small firms have become more important for contraceptive development. Although these organizations have experienced some initial difficulties, they are becoming better equipped to develop new products. Progress, however, has been slow and it is not clear whether these groups will have the resources to discover, develop, and market fundamentally new methods successfully.

Although the rate at which new products will be developed cannot be forecast precisely, significant innovations in contraceptive technology are currently being

1

studied in the United States and in other countries. Moreover, important improvements in contraception are already available to people in other countries; their appropriateness in the United States should be considered.

New methods would help men and women meet the changing needs for contraception that they face during the different stages of their reproductive lives. An increase in the total number and type of contraceptive options available would help to ensure a better, healthier match of methods to users. Furthermore, societal needs change over time, and new methods could help societies address important social problems, such as the prevalence of sexually transmitted diseases. The significant gaps that currently exist in the range of available methods could be filled, in part, by developing new, safe, effective, and acceptable contraceptive methods for men, for breastfeeding women, for teenagers, for older women, and for those with a particular health condition or illness.

Ensuring adequate and sustained financial and human resources is an important step in strengthening the ability of existing organizations and scientists to develop new contraceptives. Given the relatively small pool of scientists working in this field, the committee believes that special attention should be given to enhancing the training opportunities for young scientists interested in careers in reproduction and contraceptive development.

FDA REGULATION OF CONTRACEPTIVE PRODUCTS

The committee concludes that recent policy changes by the Food and Drug Administration (FDA) have improved the review and regulation of contraceptive products. Questions remain, however, about the standards of safety and effectiveness applied to contraceptive products. For most drugs, the FDA reviews their risks compared with their benefits against a specific health condition or illness. In the case of contraceptive products, however, the FDA assesses the potential impact of a contraceptive on *healthy* users, without sufficient recognition that the risks associated with a particular contraceptive drug or device may be outweighed by the advantages of the method for some users.

The committee believes more weight should be given to variations among potential users that could influence their contraceptive practice. In addition, the committee concludes that the FDA should increase the weight it assigns to contraceptive effectiveness and convenience of use. Given the potentially serious health consequences of an unwanted pregnancy resulting from contraceptive failure, methods with fewer side effects are not necessarily safer if they have higher failure rates. The social and health risk of pregnancy will be important considerations for users and must be weighed in the calculation of the safety of methods. The committee does not propose reducing the safety requirements applicable to contraceptives. Instead, we propose adding new criteria to the evaluation of safety to make it more specific to different groups of users.

The committee therefore proposes a change in policy with regard to FDA practices that it believes would contribute to contraceptive development: the committee recommends that the FDA further revise its procedures for evaluating new contraceptive products by recognizing special safety advantages of new methods for identifiable groups not adequately served by already approved contraceptive methods. FDA should be prepared to approve a contraceptive drug or device even if that drug or device presents a risk, *if* it can be shown that the new contraceptive also offers a safety advantage for an identifiable group of users when compared with that group's actual contraceptive practice, including nonuse. Such a contraceptive should be indicated only for a well-defined population that, in fact, is not adequately served by other contraceptives. The product's labeling should discuss all significant risks presented by the contraceptive.

The effect of such changes might be that the FDA would view as adequate to support approval a benefit-risk ratio currently viewed as inadequate to support approval. Such an approval should be subject to conditions to help ensure that approval will enhance the health of users of the new contraceptive. In order for the FDA to make an adequate assessment that a contraceptive product is beneficial, it needs feedback about its effects on the health of users. The committee's recommendation that a comprehensive postmarketing surveillance system be established is a good way to ensure systematic and timely feedback.

The committee does not consider an increase in the weight ascribed to contraceptive effectiveness and convenience to be a major change in the FDA regulation of contraceptives or a departure from the policy that the FDA applies with respect to other drugs. Rather, we view it as an effort to make the FDA's regulation of contraceptive drugs and devices more similar to its regulations of other drugs and devices. The committee strongly endorses the FDA's paramount concern for the safety of users of contraceptives, but we believe that concern can be most effectively exerted by changing the current standard applied by the FDA for approval of new contraceptives. The proposed change would still impose on contraceptive products a safety standard more demanding than that for other drugs and devices.

PRODUCTS LIABILITY LAW AFFECTING CONTRACEPTIVES

The committee also recommends a change in public policy related to liability law that would contribute to the development of new contraceptives. Two aspects of recent products liability litigation and its impact are significant in the context of contraceptives: one is the unpredictable nature of litigation, which results in part from the absence of stable and uniform national products liability rules and in part from the often erratic character of the litigation system; the other is that, although manufacturers may introduce evidence of compliance with FDA regulations in a products liability lawsuit, this evidence is given no special status in most states. FDA approval, for example, does not entitle the manufacturer to a presumption that it acted with due care. Because of the length of time necessary for development of a new contraceptive product and the costs of that development, manufacturers, in considering whether to remain in the contraceptive field, are likely to give special attention to the prospects of extensive litigation. Without changes in the products liability rules and procedures, it appears likely that even fewer firms will allocate even fewer resources to contraceptive research and development.

The committee believes that the products liability rules can be changed to remove most of their undue negative consequences for contraceptive development without increasing the health risks of contraceptive users. The committee has concluded that an aspect of a contraceptive drug or device that complies with the requirements of federal food and drug law should not be determined to be a defect or a breach of warranty under state law; that the manufacturer of that contraceptive product should not be held negligent for complying with FDA-approved designs or warnings; and therefore that the manufacturer of a specific contraceptive drug or device should not be the source of compensation to someone injured by that aspect of the particular contraceptive drug or device. This defense would not be available if the contraceptive manufacturer withheld relevant information from the FDA in the approval process, or if information developed after approval was not reviewed by the FDA for purposes of determining whether the contraceptive product, its marketing, or its labeling should be changed. The committee also notes that the important issue of providing adequate compensation to persons injured by defective products is part of a much broader question of the adequacy of existing private and social insurance mechanisms, and as such goes beyond the scope of this report.

The committee therefore recommends that Congress enact a federal products liability statute that gives contraceptive manufacturers credit for FDA approval of contraceptive drugs and devices. Pharmaceuticals and medical devices are unique among products in the United States in the degree to which quality is regulated before they are released in the market. Given that a system of careful premarketing review exists, the necessity for liability as a quality control mechanism is greatly reduced. When the FDA has considered the relevant health and safety data on a contraceptive product, has approved the product, and has required warning and instructions to accompany the product, it is sound national policy to make this approval available to manufacturers as a limited defense and not to penalize them for something they could not have known at an earlier point. Because the statute would interact with postmarketing surveillance efforts, this recommendation would be more compelling if formal postmarketing surveillance studies were generally required.

CONCLUSION

There has been a tremendous growth in the use of modern contraceptives over the past three decades. Concern about side effects and the effectiveness of existing methods and demand for safer, more effective, more convenient, and affordable contraceptives have also grown. The importance of these issues both in the United States and in other countries is likely to increase in the decades to come. But new birth control methods—even safer and more effective ones—will be of little benefit if they are not accessible, if they are not delivered properly with adequate screening and counseling, if they are not used, or if they are used incorrectly.

Better education about human reproduction, sexuality, and contraception, shared responsibility, and more open communication between partners about sex, health, and family planning are likely to increase motivation to use contraception and the ability of individuals to use methods effectively. But, unless steps are taken now to change public policy related to contraceptive development, contraceptive choice in the next century will not be appreciably different from what it is today.

1

Introduction

Most sexually active Americans have had some experience with contraception. But despite widespread contraceptive use, concern persists about the safety, effectiveness, cost, convenience, and acceptability of modern contraceptives. Outside the United States, particularly in developing countries where medical services appropriate for the diagnosis and treatment of contraceptive-related side effects are limited and where the health risks of pregnancy, labor, and delivery are much greater than in the United States, there is also a great deal of concern about people's ability to use existing contraceptive methods to meet their varying needs for safe, effective, and acceptable fertility control.

The costs of unwanted pregnancies and childbirth for mothers and children, as well as for their families and the communities in which they live, can be very high. Questions about the social costs of different patterns of fertility and the desire on the part of sexually active men and women for better contraception have led to a renewal of interest in the development of new techniques for the control of fertility. The AIDS epidemic has also focused public attention on the potential impact of new contraceptive methods, but anxiety about AIDS is just the latest in a series of factors that have led specialists and concerned citizens alike to wonder why there have been so few advances in contraceptive technology over the past several decades. This report examines the obstacles to contraceptive development as well as the opportunities that current work in the field presents.

The report addresses contraceptive development activities under way in the United States or supported by U.S. institutions. To consider the institutional arrangements and policies that influence contraceptive development in other countries would require a separate study and much greater involvement of non-American experts. There are two exceptions to our focus on the United States. First, at several places in the report, we discuss the consequences that decisions related to contraceptive development made in the United States appear to have on people in developing countries. Second, we examine the role of the World Health Organization (WHO) and its Special Programme of Research, Development, and Research Training in Human Reproduction in the development of new contraceptives. WHO is one of the most important institutions involved in contraceptive development, and American scientists and organizations have played a crucial role in WHO's program.

We hope this report will be read by the people who directly or indirectly shape contraceptive development policy in the United States. Three groups seem particularly important in this regard. First are the legislators who set policy (for example through patent and tax laws), establish budgets, earmark funds, provide direction to regulatory agencies, and otherwise act to shape research priorities for the nation. A second group we hope to reach are the executives at organizations actively involved in efforts to develop new contraceptives. This group includes people working at pharmaceutical firms, those employed by the nonprofit groups engaged in contraceptive development, as well as the staff at the National Institutes of Health, the Agency for International Development, and the private foundations that support research on new contraceptives. Third, we have tried to write the report in language and style that is easily comprehended by the public. It is a commonplace to claim that a particular problem or issue has broad public relevance, but that claim is more accurate when applied to contraceptive development than when used to describe most matters of science policy. Few other products touch so many people in so intimate and yet far-reaching ways as contraceptives do.

We have worked to provide an empirical foundation for our analysis. The committee collected and reviewed data on the prospects for the introduction of new contraceptive methods; on public attitudes toward contraceptive development; on the costs and time needed for regulatory approval of new contraceptives; on the relationships among organizations involved in contraceptive research and development; on recent and proposed changes in regulatory requirements for contraceptives; on contraceptive products liability cases; and on the availability and costs of product liability insurance for contraceptive products.

Because of the proprietary nature of information on research and development costs, new methods under development, and contraceptive products liability cases, it was impossible to obtain all of the information the committee would have liked. Individual companies were especially reluctant to divulge information on products liability cases, contraceptive sales, or research and development costs. Nevertheless, we believe the report contains ample evidence to support the committee's analysis, conclusions, and recommendations.

ORGANIZATION

The report, which is composed of nine chapters, describes the history, current status, and prospects of contraceptive development; analyzes the impact of a variety of institutional factors that shape the contraceptive development process; and makes recommendations on ways to accelerate the pace of contraceptive development in the United States.

Following this introductory chapter, Chapter 2 provides an assessment of the advantages to be gained from new contraceptive methods. We argue that new male and female contraceptive methods would contribute to the well-being of men, women, and their families both in the United States and other industrialized countries and, with potentially far greater impact, among people in the less developed world.

Chapter 3 reviews the specific contraceptive innovations that are being developed, some of which could be available within the next 15 years. Chapter 4 provides a brief overview of Americans' attitudes toward fertility control and contraceptive development, noting their roots in values related to sex, childbearing, family life, and the role of women. These values have been much debated in recent years. To the extent that government officials, researchers, and executives of U.S. drug companies see new contraceptive products as likely sources of public controversy or disapproval, development may have been discouraged.

The four chapters that follow address specific issues that the committee believes are significant influences on the pace and direction of contraceptive research and development. Chapter 5 reviews the organization of contraceptive research and development and examines how existing organizational arrangements and recent changes in them influence development. Special attention is given to the links among the various types of organizations involved in the development process and the unique problems that small firms and nonprofit organizations have in trying to bring contraceptive products to the market. Factors affecting the involvement of the pharmaceutical industry in the development and marketing of contraceptives are also discussed.

One frequently overlooked factor that may influence the speed of progress in a scientific field is the pool of scientific personnel working in the area. Chapter 6 discusses both the human and financial resources available for contraceptive research, how these have changed over time, and how these changes may have affected the pace of development.

Chapter 7 examines the role of the Food and Drug Administration (FDA) in the regulation of the development, testing, and use of contraceptives. The chapter reviews the efforts of the FDA to balance risks and benefits to individuals and society and examines recent changes in the regulation of contraceptive products. A number of specific issues related to the regulation of contraceptives in the United States and with relations between American and foreign regulatory agencies are also discussed.

Chapter 8 analyzes tort liability for contraceptive products, which many people regard as the most important barrier to development efforts in the United States. We present data on the levels and trends in liability actions for contraceptive products and review the history of cases in this area. This chapter also examines the relationship between liability and insurance, and the extent to which these affect the market for contraceptives and, hence, the incentives for research and development in this area.

The final chapter summarizes the committee's review and makes recommendations for increasing the likelihood that new contraceptives will be developed.

In most cases, when faced with a choice between summarizing and presenting the specific pieces of evidence we drew on, we chose to provide the details. We hope this will enable readers to appreciate better the complex factors that shape the contraceptive development enterprise and to better understand our arguments and recommendations. We have also provided a brief executive summary for those who wish to have an overview of the report. The report concludes with a glossary to help readers who are unfamiliar with specific technical terms.

There are no quick fixes to the problems caused by the limited range of contraceptive methods available to men and women in the United States and to millions of other men and women around the world. The regulation of human fertility is a complex process, and the development of new contraceptive products costs millions of dollars and takes years, not weeks or months, to complete. There are, however, opportunities for innovation that are not being pursued because of a series of identifiable barriers. This report analyzes those barriers, evaluates their impact on the way new contraceptives are being developed, and suggests ways of changing the organization of contraceptive development and the policies governing work in the field that we believe would accelerate the pace of development.

2

The Need for New Contraceptives

Before we discuss how new contraceptives are developed and what opportunities research offers for safer, more effective, more acceptable, more convenient, and more easily distributed products, it is important to review how current methods are used and to understand why problems of availability exist. Moreover, the case that new contraceptives would be valuable must be established. If there is little or nothing to be gained from an increase in the number and kinds of contraceptives available to men and women, there is little or nothing to be gained from further research. This chapter examines the shortcomings of existing methods, then considers how new methods might benefit the individuals using them and the societies in which they live.

An array of contraceptive methods is required to meet the varying needs of men and women at different stages of their life cycles. One method may be most appropriate for young people and those having intercourse only occasionally. Another method may be better suited to young mothers breastfeeding a first child and eager to space their pregnancies. A third method may be most appropriate for older couples who want a highly effective long-term method, because they do not want additional children but do not wish to become sterilized. Many people are not well served by currently available contraceptive methods.

With most products, we expect the normal operations of industry, the marketplace, and government policy to generate an appropriate range of product choices and speed of product development. Contraceptives, however, differ from most products in important ways. Government policies have limited the number and variety of contraceptive products available to consumers as well as the rate of contraceptive development. This situation is the result of the special characteristics of modern contraceptive methods and our orientation toward them.

Using a contraceptive benefits both the individual using the method and a variety of groups, from users' immediate families to the communities and countries in which they live. A woman benefits because contraception may contribute to her well-being by lowering the likelihood of an unwanted pregnancy and decreasing the need for abortion. Some contraceptives also help to prevent the transmission of sexually transmitted diseases. Others reduce the risk of certain cancers. Avoiding pregnancy reduces the risks of health problems associated with pregnancy and childbirth. Avoiding pregnancy may also increase a woman's ability to work outside the home. If she works, her family may benefit from the additional resources she can provide. Children's health is also improved when their mothers are able to space their pregnancies. In less developed countries, contraceptive use may contribute to slower population growth, which in turn may help promote a country's social and economic development.

The social benefits of contraception argue for public involvement in the contraceptive development process. The importance of the social dimension of population is well recognized in other areas. Because of the disparity between individual actions and state interests with respect to population, most if not all countries have policies to regulate population growth through immigration. The vast majority of less developed countries support national family planning programs to increase contraceptive use in order to reduce population growth or to improve health by enabling women to avoid high-risk and unwanted pregnancies (Lapham and Mauldin, 1987).

The committee believes the lack of an adequate array of contraceptives has adverse consequences for both individuals and for society as a whole. The inadequacy of current contraceptive methods contributes to the problems of unintended pregnancy, unwanted children, and high rates of abortions. The impact of these problems affects not only the individuals involved, but their families, friends, and the communities in which they live.

Although reducing unwanted pregnancies and abortions is a potentially important social benefit of contraception, government policies tend to devalue these and other benefits of contraceptive use for society. Most U.S. government policies toward contraception have been directed at ensuring the safe delivery of contraceptives, not at maximizing the rate of contraceptive development. Policies designed to regulate contraceptives, for example, may have impeded the rate of product development. Product reviews by the Food and Drug Administration (FDA), for example, focus on the benefits and risks to individuals and do not consider adequately the benefits to society if a contraceptive were available and used by a large number of people.

Contraceptive development has also slowed because of the difficulty of dealing with the problems posed by new technology, which require careful evaluations of complex risks and benefits. Contraceptives need to be used over an individual's reproductive lifetime: women remain fertile for about 35 years, and men even longer, and they may want to use contraception for most of that time. It is very difficult for individual users as well as for scientists and policy makers to evaluate all the risks and benefits of such long-term use in a reasonable time and at a reasonable cost. Most individuals lack the information and experience to make completely informed judgments about contraceptives, particularly regarding unknown risks and long-term effects. This limitation has been recognized in extensive government regulation involving the evaluation of product safety in many areas.

Benefits from therapeutic drugs normally are clear: a person recovers from disease (with some probability) or has a symptom relieved. The gain from contraception is no less real, but it requires use of a drug or device for a preventive purpose, frequently on a long-term basis. In addition to the benefit of reducing unwanted pregnancies and their consequences, contraceptives also have noncontraceptive health benefits. But since most people assume that contraceptive users typically are healthy at the time they contracept, these benefits involving prevention—not only of unwanted pregnancy, but of health risks associated with pregnancy—have not been sufficiently taken into account in the development of public policy. Contraceptive development has been slowed because the full individual as well as societal benefits of additional contraceptive products have not been properly recognized.

Existing public policy affects the availability of contraceptives and the rate at which new products are developed in many uncoordinated ways. Public funding supports research; government regulation controls marketing; and liability rules affect development. These and other policies help to determine the incentives to undertake research, development, and marketing of a new product. Policies affecting contraceptive development originate in different parts of government and are directed at diverse aims. It is not surprising that the complicated, uncoordinated, political, legal, and regulatory history of contraception has resulted in less than optimal progress in the development of new contraceptive methods.

These four factors—the social benefits of contraception, the complexity of contraceptive-related risks and benefits, the problems of evaluating the uncertain impact of long-term contraceptive use, and the effects of uncoordinated and sometimes discrepant public policies—interact in complex ways that the committee believes restrict the availability of contraceptive products. Although contraceptive use is widespread in the United States, many people lack access to contraceptives they consider appropriate for their particular circumstances. Every method in use today has drawbacks, and, collectively, current methods leave major gaps in the ability of people to control fertility safely, effectively, and in culturally acceptable ways throughout their reproductive life cycle. New policies could help more adequately to meet the contraceptive needs of American couples. The needs of people in developing countries for new contraceptives are even greater than those in the United States. Changes in policies that would increase contraceptive choices in less developed countries would be particularly welcome.

Although it is necessary to be concerned about the potential for abuse of users that some methods or delivery strategies present, it is also important to be concerned about the consequences of a lack of adequate methods. Limited contraceptive methods force many women and men to make difficult choices—to have an abortion or to be sterilized at a young age—that could be avoided if additional safe, effective, acceptable, and affordable contraceptives were available.

CURRENT CONTRACEPTIVE USE

Contraceptive Practice

The great social and scientific revolutions of the twentieth century have enhanced our ability to control childbearing. The vast majority of adults in the United States and several hundred million people in countries around the world have used contraceptives. Among the 54 million American women between the ages of 15 and 44 who have had intercourse, 95 percent have used contraception at some time (Forrest, 1987). Over 70 percent of all married American women of child-bearing age or their husbands currently practice contraception. In 1987 the pill was the single most popular contraceptive method in the United States, followed by female sterilization, condoms, and vasectomies (Forrest and Fordyce, 1988). Never before in history has a systemic drug such as the oral contraceptive been used so widely on a continuing basis by predominantly healthy women for a preventive purpose.

Before describing the potential advantages of new contraceptive methods, it is useful to review currently available contraceptives. Table 2.1 provides an overview of contraceptive methods available in the United States; the table includes information on prevalence of use and failure rates as well as a brief account of the methods' major advantages and disadvantages. It is important to note that failure rates, i.e., the rate of accidental pregnancy in the first year of use, include both user failure—failure to use the method properly as well as lack of consistent use—and method failure.

About a fifth of all women ages 18 to 49 exposed to the risk of unintended pregnancy have been sterilized. The advantages of sterilization are its high effectiveness and the fact that a single procedure provides complete protection with very little health risk. The permanence of sterilization and the difficulty of reversing the procedure, however, are disadvantages for some people. Female sterilization requires a skilled medical practitioner and, although complications are rare, they are not unheard of.

Vasectomy provides protection for about 15 percent of the partners of the women exposed to the risk of unintended pregnancy. Like female sterilization, vasectomy is a permanent method in which a single procedure provides long-term protection against pregnancy with an extremely low risk of negative health effects. Like female sterilization, reversal of vasectomy is possible but successful only on a limited basis.

Oral contraceptives are used by about one-third of those exposed to the risk of unintended pregnancy. The pill contains synthetic hormones that stop ovulation by interfering with cyclical hormonal changes. The pill is easily used. In addition to being easy to use, the pill causes regular menstrual periods, protects against ectopic pregnancy, and reduces the risk of certain pelvic infections as well as ovarian and uterine cancer. The pill's disadvantages include minor side effects and more serious problems such as a greater risk among oral contraceptive users of developing blood clots, heart attacks, and strokes. The risk of a heart attack or stroke is especially high for users over 35 who smoke or who have high blood pressure. About 3 percent of the women who use the pill will become pregnant accidentally during the first year of use.

In the United States, the intrauterine device (IUD) is used by 3 percent of women exposed to the risk of unintended pregnancy. The IUD is a much more popular method in some other countries. Although the process by which IUDs prevent pregnancy is still unclear, when placed in the uterus they are believed to induce an unsuitable environment for both eggs and sperm. The advantages of IUDs are their long-term protection, their reversibility, and the fact that, once inserted, they do not require frequent attention. Insertion requires a skilled medical practitioner, and IUDs may cause increased bleeding or spotting, cramping, and pain. Perforation of the uterus occurs in about 1 in 2,500 insertions. The most serious complication associated with IUD use is an increased risk of pelvic inflammatory disease among women with more than one sexual partner. Accidental failure rates during the first year of IUD use average 6 percent.

The condom is used by 16 percent of the partners of women, ages 18 to 49, exposed to the risk of unintended pregnancy. And 12 percent of women whose partners use condoms will become pregnant accidentally in the first year of use. The condom is easy to use, inexpensive, and does not require a prescription. Its greatest advantage may be that it protects against sexually transmitted diseases, including AIDS. Some people believe the condom and other barrier methods interfere with sexual relations.

The diaphragm is used by 4–6 percent of contraceptors. Two large clinic-based studies in which women had proper training in diaphragm use had failure rates of about 2 percent (Vessey et al., 1982; Lane et al., 1976). Several smaller clinic-based studies had failure rates of 11 to 13 percent (Malyk and Kompare, 1983; Edelman, 1983). Population-based studies have had the highest rates—up to 23 percent (Ryder, 1973; Schirm et al., 1982). The diaphragm offers some protection against sexually transmitted diseases and pelvic inflammatory disease and possibly cervical cancer.

The remaining methods—the contraceptive sponge, withdrawal, periodic abstinence, vaginal foams, creams, and jellies—have failure rates of between 18 and 21 percent. The advantages of these methods include their availability

TABLE 2.1 Characteristics and Effectiveness of Contraceptive Methods Generally Available in the United States

Method	Estimated % Use Among Contraceptors	% Accidental Pregnancy in the 1st Year of Use	What It Is and How It Works	Advantages	Disadvantages
Male sterilization (vasectomy)	14	.15	Permanent method in which the vas deferens, through which the sperm travel from the testes to the penis, is cut and blocked so that sperm can no longer enter the semen.	Single procedure; no subsequent health or safety risks; failure of procedure is very rare.	Requires skilled medical practitioner; minor complications including swelling & pain are common; blood clots, infection, & epididymitis occur in 1-2% of patients; death from infection can occur but is very rare; procedures should be considered permanent, although with skilled microsurgical techniques it can be reversed in about 50% of cases.
Female sterilization	19	.4	Permanent method of contraception in which the fallopian tubes are occluded so that the egg and sperm cannot meet. The tubes are surgically closed with bands, clips, electrocautery, or by cutting and tying. Laparoscopy, minilaparotomy, and postpartum laparotomy are the surgical procedures used.	Single procedure; little health or safety risk; failure of procedure is rare.	Requires skilled medical practitioner; complications are rare (bleeding, infection, injury to other organs, anesthesia complications); death can occur but is very rare; reversibility is limited and requires abdominal microsurgical procedure in skilled hands.
Combined (estrogen and progestin) oral contraceptive pill (OC)	32	3	The oral contraceptive pill combines synthetic forms of the hormones progesterone and estrogen. Stops ovulation by interfering with cyclical	Easily used; reduces about 50% of the risk of certain pelvic infections; decreases risk of ovarian and	OCs have an inhibiting effect on lactation. Failure rate increases if the pill is not taken regularly; common side effects include breast tenderness, nausea,

Method			Description	Benefits	Side effects
Oral contraceptive pill (OC), progestin-only (minipill)	(Unavailable for minipill.)	5	hormonal changes required for ovulation. Pills are taken every day in 21-day cycles (or 28-day cycles, with 7 placebo tablets). The minipill contains progestin only. It is taken continuously and causes thickening of the cervical mucus, decreasing its penetrability to spermatozoa. It produces atrophy of the endometrium, interfering with implantation. It also may inhibit ovulation.	uterine cancer by approximately 50% compared with nonusers of OCs; causes regular painless menstrual periods with decreased blood loss (may help or correct anemia); protects against ectopic pregnancy, benign cystic breast disease, and ovarian cysts. The minipill does not affect lactation; does not cause the OC-related side effects, high blood pressure, and headaches.	depression, headache, vomiting, weight gain or loss, spotting between periods. Earlier high-dose OCs were associated with a greater risk of cardiovascular diseases such as blood clots, heart attacks, & strokes; risk of heart attack & stroke increases for users over age 35 who smoke, and/or have high blood pressure. OC users have a greater risk than nonusers of developing gall bladder symptoms, but only during first year of use. The minipill has a higher pregnancy rate than combined OCs; is more likely to cause menstrual irregularity and vaginal bleeding.
Intrauterine device (IUD)	3	6	Small plastic device placed in the uterus that is believed to induce an unsuitable environment for both eggs and sperm, but the process is still unclear. The two available IUDs in the United States include Progestasert, which releases progesterone and is replaced yearly, and Cu-T 380A, which contains copper and is replaced every 4 years.	Single procedure provides effective long-term protection; progesterone-releasing IUDs decrease bleeding in contrast to other IUDs.	Insertion requires trained health care practitioner; common side effects include increased bleeding or spotting, cramping, and pain; perforation occurs in about 1/2,500 insertions; pregnancy while an IUD is in place may be ectopic or result in a septic spontaneous abortion—both potentially life-threatening; pelvic inflammatory disease (PID) is a rare but

TABLE 2.1 Continued

Method	Estimated % Use Among Contraceptors	% Accidental Pregnancy in the 1st Year of Use	What It Is and How It Works	Advantages	Disadvantages
					serious complication, seen most commonly as a result of a sexually transmitted disease. PID rarer among women in monogamous relationships.
Condom	17	12	Sheath of thin rubber (latex) that is placed on the erect penis to collect semen and to prevent sperm from entering the vagina.	Easy to use; inexpensive; does not require a prescription; protects against sexually transmitted diseases, including AIDS.	Condoms deteriorate and are ineffective when stored in too much heat, humidity, or sunlight and may tear if roughly handled.
Diaphragm	4–6	2–23[a]	Soft rubber cup that covers the cervix. Contraceptive cream or jelly is placed in the diaphragm before intercourse.	Protects against certain sexually transmitted diseases and cervical cancer; can be used safely by nursing mothers.	Women who use the diaphragm may be more prone to bladder infections; allergic reaction to rubber or cream or jelly is possible; diaphragm may dislodge during sexual intercourse; diaphragm must be cleaned and checked for weak spots and holes; requires fitting by a trained health care worker; not recommended for women with poor vaginal muscle tone.
Contraceptive sponge	3	18	Synthetic substance that is soft, round, and impregnated with spermicide. The sponge is	Does not require prescription; may protect against certain	Removal problems may occur; may cause an allergic reaction; risk of pregnancy is higher than

Method		Description		Advantages	Disadvantages
		inserted into the vagina before sexual intercourse, where it releases spermicide. The sponge is for one time use only over a 24-hour period and should never be reused.		sexually transmitted diseases.	with other reversible methods; possible risk of toxic shock reported.
Natural fertility control (forms of periodic abstinence)	4	Requires the couple to refrain from sexual intercourse during the fertile period of a woman's menstrual cycle. The most common ways used to determine the approximate time of ovulation and the fertile period include the calendar, temperature, and cervical mucus methods.	20	Requires no drugs.	Risk of pregnancy is high; requires high motivation of both sexual partners.
Vaginal contraceptives	2	Foams, creams, jellies, tablets, and suppositories that contain spermicides and are inserted into the vagina before intercourse. They inactivate sperm and mechanically prevent sperm from entering the uterus.	21	Do not require prescription; may protect against certain sexually transmitted diseases; may be used by any woman unless she is allergic to the product.	Relatively unreliable and must be used 5-10 minutes before each act of intercourse; may produce slight genital irritation.

[a]Training and proper use are critical; see text.
Source: This table is a modified version of the Population Crisis Committee's chart "A Guide to Modern Contraceptive Methods" (April 1987). Contraceptive prevalence figures are from Forrest and Fordyce (1988). Contraceptive failure rates are from Trussell and Kost (1987).

without prescription and the lack of serious side effects, independent of those associated with their relatively high failure rates. These methods are not very popular in the United States. Withdrawal and periodic abstinence are each used by about 5 percent of those exposed to the risk of unintended pregnancy; foams, creams, and jellies and tablets and suppositories by about 1 percent of those exposed to the risk of pregnancy. In some other countries, methods not approved for use in the United States are available. These methods are described briefly in Chapter 3.

The large number of people who practice contraception have different desires, values, and needs, which can be met best by a variety of contraceptive methods. Not only do people differ in what they like and dislike, but individuals' contraceptive needs also change during their reproductive lifetimes. The needs of adolescents are different from an adult's need for child spacing or for termination of childbearing. People's health differs, as does their reaction to different contraceptive products. Because people live under diverse social, economic, and cultural conditions and are served by a wide variety of health care systems, they need different methods of contraception. Although a variety of contraceptive methods exists, the committee believes that substantial gaps remain in the array of methods available for particular groups.

The importance that couples in the United States give to effective contraception and the problems they encounter with existing methods are illustrated by the large proportion of couples who are surgically sterilized. Fifteen or more years after their first marriage, 44 percent of all women practicing contraception are sterilized, and another 24 percent are married to men who are sterilized. These figures confirm that at some point American women are ready to stop childbearing. These data also suggest that there are problems with available temporary methods.

Given the absence of acceptable alternative choices and the problems with existing contraceptive technology, women may seek sterilization earlier than they might otherwise choose. The side effects of existing methods and concern about potential problems discourage long-term use of the most modern temporary methods. Since the likelihood of experiencing a serious adverse side effect with the pill increases with age, older women are more likely to look for an alternative method. Indeed, the pill is used by almost half of all contracepting newlyweds, but its use falls steadily as women's age and duration of marriage increases. Given the low family size goals characteristic of couples in the United States, they want a highly effective method. For many of them, surgical sterilization is the chosen alternative. The available data suggest, however, that regret at being sterilized is not uncommon. One review found between 2 and 13 percent of the sterilized women surveyed between 6 months and 6 years following sterilization expressed regret; between 1 and 3 percent underwent reversal (Lee et al., 1989). Requests for surgical repair of sterilization are increasing, particularly among women sterilized in their twenties or early thirties (Grubb et al., 1985). Estimates suggest that as many as 5 to 8 percent of all sterilized women seek surgical repair (Henry et al., 1980).

Women in the United States are not alone in their desire for effective contraception. Worldwide, about a half billion women are currently using some method of contraception; an estimated three-quarters of these women live in the less developed world (United Nations, 1987a). Although their choice of methods may vary from country to county, the vast majority of married women in Western industrialized countries practice contraception. In most Western European countries, for example, between 70 and 85 percent of all women ages 15 to 49 use contraception (United Nations, 1987a). In developing countries, contraceptive practice ranges from only 1 percent of currently married couples in some African countries to over 60 percent in such Asian and Latin American countries as Thailand, South Korea, Panama, and Costa Rica (Mauldin and Segal, 1986).

In many less developed countries, the proportion of women practicing contraception is lower than in the industrialized countries, but contraceptives are employed by a large and typically growing number of women. In the newly industrialized countries, levels of contraceptive practice are similar to those in the United States and Western Europe. In Korea, for example, 70 percent of all married women of reproductive age use contraception. Even in some of the poorer developing countries, contraceptive use is widespread. Over a third of married Indian women of reproductive age currently use a contraceptive, as do 30 percent of those in Egypt (United Nations, 1987a). Despite the increase in contraceptive prevalence in some countries, high failure rates and high discontinuation resulting from the use of inappropriate methods of contraception indicate that better delivery systems and more effective, safe, and affordable contraceptive options are needed.

The safety, effectiveness, and acceptability of contraceptives are particularly important for the many women who use them, since women bear the greatest burden of contraceptive side effects. The available contraceptive choices limit the ability of men, who might otherwise do so, to effectively share responsibility for contraception with their female partners. The number of American men who use condoms or who have had vasectomies suggests that many men are willing to share the responsibility for contraceptive practice, thus reducing periods of exposure to the risks of contraceptive use for a partner who otherwise would bear the full responsibility and the full risk.

Several groups of women, particularly older women and those with chronic diseases, need contraception but are unsuitable or poor candidates for the most highly effective contraceptives now available. Women with insulin-dependent diabetes or those with certain types of cardiovascular disease, for example, are not good candidates for either hormonal or intrauterine contraception. New methods that do not aggravate systemic diseases and do not increase the risk of infection would be of great benefit to these women.

Contraceptive Effectiveness

Although existing contraceptive technology can be highly effective, the situation is not as bright as most people, including most users, believe. One recent review of research on contraceptive effectiveness summarized the current situation: "Despite the fact that most methods do well if used consistently and correctly, failure rates in actual use are generally not low. A contraceptive that is inexpensive, is easy to use, has few side effects, and is highly efficacious is still needed" (Trussell and Kost, 1987:272).

The data available on contraceptive effectiveness, shown in Table 2.1, indicate the range of effectiveness with which contraceptive methods are used. (Failure rates are expressed in terms of the percentage of women using a method who become pregnant accidently during the first year of use.) The studies from which the data came were conducted mainly in the United States. Evidence from both developed and less developed countries (Laing, 1978; Thapa et al., 1988) indicates that the actual effectiveness of temporary methods of contraception varies among different groups within a country. Effectiveness is higher among better educated women and among those who want no more children. To the extent that a larger proportion of the users of a particular method in a developing country are likely to be less well educated about contraception, the effectiveness of a particular method will be lower.

The effectiveness of different contraceptive methods varies widely. Fewer than one half of one percent of the users of sterilization in the United States will experience an accidental pregnancy in the first year of use. The comparable figure for oral contraceptives is 3 percent; for the intrauterine device (IUD), 6 percent; for the condom, 12 percent; for the diaphragm, the cervical cap, and withdrawal, up to 18 percent. Of the women who use spermicides, the contraceptive sponge, or who practice periodic abstinence as a means of fertility control, 20 percent or more will become pregnant within the first year of use (Trussell and Kost, 1987).

The failure rates, which may sound small, can have a substantial impact, especially, of course, on the women who become pregnant and on their partners. In 1987 an estimated 6.9 million American men used condoms as a method of contraception. If the average annual accidental pregnancy rate is 8 percent (lower than the 12 percent for the first year because users learn to use their method of choice more effectively over time, and less effective users tend to stop using the method), there would be over 500,000 accidental pregnancies in the United States each year because of the low effectiveness of the condom in actual use. Using data from the 1987 Ortho survey of married and unmarried women currently protected by various contraceptive methods and several estimates of method-specific contraceptive failure, we estimate that between 1.2 and 3.0 million accidental pregnancies occurred in 1987 as a result of contraceptive failure (Forrest and Fordyce, 1988). It is most likely that the actual number is between

1.6 and 2.0 million. Many of these accidental pregnancies result in abortion. Forrest and Silverman (1988) estimate that about half of the approximately 1.5 million abortions performed in the United States each year are the result of contraceptive failure.

An important, although not well-studied, determinant of contraceptive effectiveness is the quality of the system that delivers family planning services (Bruce, 1987). People who are well informed about the side effects they will experience and who understand how to use a method properly practice contraception more effectively than those who are not properly informed. Indeed, the availability of health personnel, clinics, or pharmacies may determine the effectiveness with which contraception can be practiced. Even simple matters such as resupply cannot be taken for granted in the rural areas of many less developed countries. There are rarely sufficient resources to provide people with the information and support they need for the most effective use of existing methods. New methods that are simpler, safer, and more convenient to use could make the task of providing information, education, and services easier and less of a drain on the financial and human resources of the service delivery systems of developing countries.

POTENTIAL EFFECTS OF NEW CONTRACEPTIVES

Reducing Abortions

Low birth rates and a low level of unwanted childbearing can be achieved by less effective contraceptive methods, if women obtain abortions when contraceptive failure occurs. The stronger the desire to reduce abortion, the greater should be the investment to develop new methods of contraception. The effects of new methods would vary among populations depending on their levels of fertility and patterns of fertility control. In industrialized nations, in which fertility is already low, the greatest impact of new methods would probably be to reduce the number of abortions and to provide couples with a better array of fertility control options. In developing countries with high birth rates, the greatest impact of new methods would be to reduce the number of births. However, to the extent that new contraceptive methods reduced unsafe abortions in developing countries, they would also help lower maternal mortality. Recent studies have found that between 5 and 30 percent of maternal deaths in developing countries are abortion-related (Lettenmaier et al., 1988). Increased contraceptive use and more effective contraceptive practice could help reduce unsafe abortions and the complications and deaths associated with them (Viel, 1985).

One recent analysis of the potential impact of improved contraception in six European countries concluded that a reduction in contraceptive failures would result in a 5- to 10-percent reduction in pregnancies. However, if the new methods increased the overall level of contraceptive use and thus reduced the occurrence of unwanted pregnancy, a further reduction of one-third to one-half of all abortions would result (Westoff et al., 1987).

Contraception and Health

A large volume of evidence from countries at all stages of development and with a variety of health care systems indicates that using contraception to space births and to terminate childbearing is safer for women and their children than unregulated childbearing (Lee et al., 1989). The contribution new contraceptive methods may make to improved health for women and their children provides an important justification for investments in this field.

Even in the United States, for women under the age of 35, not using a contraceptive is associated with a higher mortality than employing any contraceptive method, including use of the pill by women who smoke (Ory et al., 1983). Contraceptive side effects pose a much more serious risk in poor countries, where diagnosis and treatment are frequently inadequate and problems resulting from untreated illness may have far more serious repercussions. New methods that make possible safer contraceptive practice would provide important health benefits to men and women around the world.

According to one estimate (World Health Organization, 1986a), the number of women who die each year from pregnancy-related causes may be as high as 500,000, all but 6,000 or so of them in less developed countries. According to one recent study, if all unwanted pregnancies were avoided, between 25 and 40 percent of all maternal deaths would also be avoided (Maine and Rosenfield, 1982). To the extent that new methods would increase contraceptive use and effectiveness, they could significantly improve women's health.

Children may also benefit when their mothers are able to control their fertility. Children born at least 2 years apart have lower rates of infant death than those born closer together. If new methods help to reduce births in high-risk categories of maternal age or birth order or among women with short birth intervals, then infant and childhood mortality might decline as the new contraceptives become more popular (Hobcraft, 1987; Trussell and Pebley, 1984; National Research Council, 1989).

Reducing the Problems Associated With Existing Methods

Although the risks of currently approved contraceptive methods are on balance lower than those of pregnancy, in a small fraction of users the health consequences of some current contraceptives are serious. There are health complications and rare deaths associated with existing methods, even though these can be reduced to a minimum in properly screened women. New contraceptives may have fewer side effects and complications than those associated with the existing methods and thereby add to the attractiveness and safety of contraceptive practice.

The major reason given by American women for not contracepting is fear of complications (Ory et al., 1983). Side effects are offered as a major reason for discontinuing pill use by women in many countries (Janowitz et al., 1986; Stephen and Chamratrithirong, 1988). Women discontinuing pill use for health reasons often switch to less effective methods (Janowitz et al., 1986).

Nausea, breast enlargement, weight gain, loss of libido, and dizziness are the most common complaints of oral contraceptive users. But more serious complications, such as cardiovascular problems that require hospitalization, also occur among pill users. Although the evidence regarding the link between the pill and breast cancer is conflicting, the uncertainty of the relationship has caused concern among many women. The limited popularity of the IUD in the United States no doubt is due in part to its perceived association with an increased risk of pelvic inflammatory disease (PID) and infertility. Although rare, perforation of the uterus is another potentially serious complication of IUD use.

The natural family planning methods have no side effects, but their effectiveness is low relative to other methods. Periodic abstinence or the daily testing of body temperature or cervical mucus are viewed by many women as a major inconvenience. The procedures these methods require reduce the acceptability of the natural methods for many couples and the effectiveness with which they are practiced.

Although sterilization is generally a very safe operation in the United States, major complications of sterilization procedures include unintended major surgery to control bleeding, rehospitalization because of pelvic infection, vaginal bleeding, and urinary tract infections. Deaths resulting from sterilization are very rare; the major cause of death is complications resulting from the use of general anesthesia, not the sterilization procedure itself. Vasectomy is safer than female sterilization and has few complications or postoperative hospitalizations associated with it, even in the developing world.

Barrier methods—condoms, diaphragms, foams, jellies, creams, suppositories, sponges—do not have serious side effects. Moreover, barrier methods carry an important health benefit—the prevention of sexually transmitted diseases. However, failure rates for barrier methods and periodic abstinence are significantly higher than those for the pill, the IUD, and sterilization. Thus women using these methods have a greater likelihood of becoming pregnant and thus of being exposed to the risks associated with childbirth.

The health hazards of existing contraceptive methods are usually due to a mismatch between the method and the user. Cardiovascular complications of oral contraceptives, for example, are not a significant risk for young nonsmokers. The risk of PID is higher among IUD users with several sexual partners. The availability of a wider range of contraceptive methods would improve the matching of methods and users. Fewer people would have to use methods that are not acceptable or appropriate for their health status or life-style.

Increasing the Coverage and Quality of Contraceptive Services

New contraceptive methods may also help increase the coverage and quality of contraceptive services, particularly in developing countries. Of the countries that adopted official policies to provide support for family planning programs, all but India did so after the pill and IUD became available in the early 1960s (Greep et al., 1976). The provision of government support for family planning services was part of the post-World War II modernization process. As such, it required a new political and social environment, not simply a new contraceptive technology. But it is also true that the limitations of then-existing contraceptive methods were so extensive that many government leaders were discouraged from undertaking family planning programs. Bernard Berelson noted the importance of the introduction of the IUD for family planning programs in the 1960s: "By giving national programs some hope of success . . . [the IUD] stimulated a wholly new level of effort, improved the morale of family planning workers from the top down and, most importantly, brought about the development of family planning organizations in a form and magnitude not previously known" (Berelson, 1969:365).

The experience of several national family planning programs in developing countries demonstrates that additional couples begin to practice contraception each time a new method is introduced (Freedman and Berelson, 1976; Fathalla, 1989). A new method—an injectable contraceptive—recently had this effect in Bangladesh (Phillips et al., 1989). Although some users of new methods are drawn from the pool of women using existing methods, the available evidence suggests that new methods attract new users.

There are populations, even in the United States, to whom very few of the existing available methods are acceptable. Scrimshaw et al. (1987), in a study of low-income Hispanic women in Los Angeles, found that those who were breastfeeding and who wished to space their children were without adequate contraception. They hesitated to take the pill because of its possible impact on lactation, and they found barrier methods unacceptable to themselves or their partners. It is possible that the situation among this group is a prologue to what will happen for increasingly larger groups of women in the United States as contraceptive choices become more limited at least in part because of the withdrawal of contraceptive products from the market by major pharmaceutical firms.

The problems are not only those of the low-income community. U.S. couples in their twenties and thirties complain about the lack of appropriate methods. Women in this group who cannot or do not want to use oral contraceptives and are not ready to be sterilized must rely on less effective barrier methods, periodic abstinence, withdrawal, or a limited selection of IUDs—providing, of course, that they are not removed from the market.

None of the currently available methods is well suited for the immediate postpartum period. The IUD, which does not interfere with lactation, can be inserted immediately postpartum or at the time of hospital discharge, but rates of expulsion, perforation, and unintended pregnancy are higher than when the IUD is inserted at any other time. Progestin-only oral contraceptives (sometimes called "minipills") have been recommended for postpartum use, as have subdermal implants such as NORPLANT® (see Chapter 3). However, until more information on the long-term follow-up is available, the potential risk of synthetic hormone transfer to the baby is a cause of concern regarding the use of these methods.

THE IMPORTANCE OF CONTRACEPTIVE DELIVERY

Accounts of the large number of people in need of family planning services warrant the question of whether and to what extent this unmet need could best be served by better delivery of existing contraceptive methods. Some analysts have claimed that the problem of contraceptive use is not a so-called hardware problem, but a software problem (Djerassi, 1981). From this point of view, the need for better, more available contraceptives can best be served by improvements in delivery systems rather than by the development of new products. In many developing countries, the problems with delivery systems are particularly acute. Certainly, improved delivery would help and, for the immediate future, it is the only alternative. But the need to better deliver the contraceptive methods that are available should not lead one to underestimate the potential impact of new, safer, and more convenient techniques. The introduction of new methods could stimulate an expansion in the delivery system in part because, if health and family planning program managers have something new to sell or offer, they may be encouraged to expand their outlets.

New methods could influence fertility in several ways—by increasing safety (yielding fewer adverse effects) and effectiveness (yielding fewer pregnancies), increasing acceptability and use (yielding more users), or increasing continuation (producing longer durations of use). Because most modern methods of contraception are relatively effective, the impact of new methods will probably come from greater acceptance, longer periods of use, or both. If 30 percent of the population at risk uses a method of contraception (about the current level of contraceptive practice in Egypt or Bolivia), then a 10-point increase in the average continuation of use (that is, a 10-percent increase in the number using the method for a full year) would have the same demographic impact as about a 4.5 percentage point increase in contraceptive prevalence. If continuation rates were 90 percent during the first year of use instead of the 50 to 70 percent for most temporary methods, it would make a substantial difference (Berelson, 1978).

It is important, however, not to exaggerate the impact that new technology would have. A plausible case can be made that improved delivery of existing methods could also make a large difference in acceptance rates. The lowest contraceptive prevalence is typically found in countries with the weakest family planning programs (Lapham and Mauldin, 1987:671). Moreover, the experience of family planning programs in developing countries such as those in Indonesia and Thailand suggests that large increases in contraceptive use and corresponding declines in fertility are possible with current methods. Moreover, one possibility is that in some countries, for example those in sub-Saharan Africa, the demand for contraception is so low that neither improvements in contraceptive technology nor better delivery of services would encourage significantly greater use in the short term.

Nevertheless, the contribution of new contraceptive methods to an improvement in the coverage and impact of family planning programs is likely to be particularly important in the less developed world. In a large and growing number of countries, access to family planning services is considered a basic human right, similar to good health or literacy. There is little debate about the desirability of programs to provide couples with access to easy, affordable, and effective means of family planning.

CONCLUSION

New methods would help couples meet the changing needs for contraception that they face during different stages of their reproductive lives. An increase in the total number and type of contraceptive options available would help to ensure a better, healthier match of methods to users. Furthermore, societal needs change over time, and new methods could help societies address important social problems. In recent years in the United States, for example, the pattern of premarital intercourse has changed, as has exposure to sexually transmitted diseases. To the extent that such social changes take place, the need for contraceptive methods is altered. In this respect, then, contraception is not like other aspects of preventive medicine. One polio vaccine solved the problem of poliomyelitis, but one contraceptive will never meet all societies' and all individuals' changing needs for fertility regulation (Potts and Lincoln, 1988). There are important and obvious gaps in the range of available methods. These gaps could be filled, in part, by developing new, safe, effective, and acceptable methods for men, for breastfeeding women, for teenagers, for older women, and for those with particular health conditions.

There is no simple, straightforward account of the likely impact of new contraceptive methods on fertility and health. Human reproduction and its control are elements in a very complex system of multiple interactive variables, which change over time, vary from place to place, and affect people differently. It is difficult to measure the importance of a new contraceptive method relative to improvements in delivery systems, to increased information about existing methods, to changes in the status of women, or in the motivation to control fertility. New methods of contraception are not a panacea for all the problems associated with unwanted pregnancy and childbirth around the world. Nor should the development of new methods be viewed as a substitute for improving the delivery of existing products and increasing education about sexuality, human reproduction, and family planning. Greater attention must also be given to the factors that promote contraceptive use among individuals seeking to avoid pregnancy. Better education about human reproduction, sexuality, and contraception, shared responsibility, and more open communication between partners about sex, health, and contraception are likely to increase motivation to use contraception and the ability of individuals to use methods effectively. Without the proper motivation, knowledge, and communication among potential users, new and improved contraceptive methods may gain only limited acceptance or may be used improperly.

More attention should also be given to developing new contraceptive methods. We must work to improve the technology used by couples to plan their families. New methods are needed to help reduce the level of unwanted pregnancy, the use of abortion, and the health risks of childbearing. The committee believes that the important societal and individual benefits of safe and effective contraceptive use argue strongly for a larger number and greater variety of contraceptives.

3

The Current Status of
Contraceptive Research

Since the introduction of the pill and the IUD in the early 1960s, no fundamentally new contraceptive methods have been approved for use in the United States. This chapter discusses the new contraceptive methods currently being studied both in the United States and abroad. We try to provide an overview of promising scientific leads, and thus of methods that the public might reasonably expect to be available within the next 10 to 15 years. Unfortunately, such a general criterion is hard to apply without dispute. One person's promising new development is, for another, a preposterous idea or only a trivial modification. We have chosen to be inclusive rather than exclusive, since our aim is to provide a sense of what might be possible if the barriers to faster development were reduced. We have also included a brief overview of important modifications of existing methods to enable readers to evaluate more knowledgeably the range of potential innovations that changes in public policies could yield.

RESEARCH LEADS

Dramatic changes in the range of available contraceptive technology are unlikely to occur in the 1990s (Djerassi, 1987; Harper, 1983). Most of the contraceptive methods that will be available in the United States between now and the turn of the century will constitute modest improvements to existing methods. So, although no single new contraceptive will be a panacea for the fertility control needs of all people, scientists are studying a number of promising leads that could result in the development of contraceptives that have few side effects and health risks and are more effective, more easily administered and used, and less costly.

30

The acceptability of new methods or of modifications of existing methods among potential users and their effect on nonuse are difficult to predict. Advocates of new technology often exaggerate the potential impact of innovations, while critics of new methods often underestimate the likely influence of such changes. Modest improvements in existing methods will probably not significantly increase acceptability and use. But major changes, such as that made possible by a contraceptive implant, could substantially increase the acceptability of contraceptive practice.

It is extremely difficult to estimate when a particular new contraceptive will be available. The entire development process is surrounded by the uncertainties of scientific research, funding, marketing feasibility, and regulatory approval. Based on a 1980 survey of contraceptive development experts, the congressional Office of Technology Assessment (OTA) named nine fertility control methods as "highly likely before 1990" (OTA, 1981). Only three of these technologies—triphasic pills, the Copper T380A intrauterine device, and the Today contraceptive sponge— were available in the United States as of June 1989. Two steroidal methods, long-acting injections (e.g., Depo-Provera) and implants (e.g., NORPLANT®), are available in other countries. (A New Drug Application for NORPLANT® to be used in the United States has been filed with the FDA.) Four methods—improved ovulation-detection methods, vaginal rings, luteinizing hormone-releasing hormone (LHRH), and prostaglandin analogues—are being studied but will not be available in the near future. None of the 11 technologies designated by OTA as "possible by 1990 but prospects doubtful" is likely to be available for several years, and some could take an additional decade or longer to be developed or could, indeed, not be developed at all.

Given the problems encountered in previous efforts to identify the range of potential new contraceptives, we do not argue strongly for our list of possible contraceptive innovations. Instead, we want to emphasize that significant developments are possible and are being studied and that, in some cases, couples in other countries are already benefiting from new methods not yet available in the United States. Each new method represents possible improvement over existing methods, either because of new drugs or materials or because of a more effective, safer, or more convenient mode of administration. Because some of the methods being studied use drugs or other substances already approved by the FDA, the approval process for them may be less cumbersome, time-consuming, and costly than for a totally new method.

Female Methods

New methods of delivering contraceptive steroids are being evaluated in clinical trials, and some are expected to be available for general use during the 1990s. These new delivery systems include injections, implants, transdermal patches (through the skin), vaginal suppositories and rings, and sublingual tablets (under the tongue). Because most of the new delivery systems release the drug into the bloodstream at a constant and slower rate and in smaller doses than existing oral contraceptives, they may have fewer adverse health effects than the pill. Such delivery systems are also more convenient for some users than oral tablets.

In addition to the injectables already available in other countries, new formulations of *injectables using microspheres and microcapsules* are undergoing human trials and may become available by the early to mid-1990s, assuming there are no major problems or delays in clinical testing (Liskin and Blackburn, 1987). Similar in concept to time-released cold capsules, these injectables consist of one or more hormones encased in biodegradable capsules and suspended in a sterile solution. The capsules release hormones gradually to block ovulation. Depending on the formulation, one injection can provide contraception for one, three, or six months. The most promising microspheres contain one of the progestins, norethindrone (NET) or norgestimate. A disadvantage of this approach is that, once administered, it cannot be removed or reversed.

Injectable microspheres with NET have been tested in nearly 200 women, and more extensive clinical trials are under way (Beck and Pope, 1984; Rivera et al., 1984; Liskin and Blackburn, 1987). The pregnancy rate is expected to be similar to that of oral contraceptives, but the incidence of side effects may be lower. Irregular menstrual bleeding and the absence of menses are the main side effects found in the clinical trials to date.

Two formulations of progestin-estrogen combination once-a-month injectable contraceptives have been developed by the World Health Organization's Special Programme in Human Reproduction. A large Phase III multicenter study has been completed and has confirmed their high efficacy as well as the regular vaginal bleeding patterns associated with their use. Plans are being made for introductory field studies in Latin America and Southeast Asia.

Biodegradable pellets are similar to the new silastic contraceptive implants (see below), in that they are a long-acting, slow-release contraceptive. But unlike the implant, the pellets can be removed only within the first few months of insertion. The rice-size pellets, which are inserted under the skin in the hip or upper arm, slowly release progestins, thereby inhibiting conception. The pellets themselves are absorbed while the hormones are being released. The two types of pellets currently undergoing clinical trials are effective for one to one and a half years. The main side effect identified to date is irregular menstrual bleeding, particularly in the first few months of use (Program for Applied Research on Fertility Regulation, 1985). It is estimated that they could be available for general use in the mid-1990s. The inability to remove the pellets, once administered, is a disadvantage.

The *vaginal ring* consists of a silicone rubber ring about the size of a diaphragm that continuously releases steroids to suppress ovulation and thicken the cervical mucus, thereby preventing sperm from entering the uterus. Vaginal rings have the advantage of being user-controlled and readily reversible. Depending on their formulation, vaginal rings are worn continuously for three months and then replaced, or for three weeks at a time and then removed for one week to allow monthly bleeding. The rings may be removed for a few hours without reducing their effectiveness and do not need to be in place during intercourse (Harper, 1983). Vaginal rings do not need to be specially fitted, but first-time users should be screened and instructed in proper use.

Research is most advanced on a continuous-wear vaginal ring containing levonorgestrel, the same progestin used in some oral contraceptives. However, the pregnancy rate observed in clinical trials of the ring was higher than that of oral contraceptives. In one trial involving about 1,000 women, there were 3.5 pregnancies per 100 woman-years of use (WHO, 1985b). Similar to other progestin-only methods, the main side effect associated with the levonorgestrel vaginal ring is irregular menstrual patterns. Clinical trials have been completed, and an application for marketing approval in the United Kingdom has been submitted. Introductory studies are expected to follow validation of the ring's manufacturing process. Other vaginal rings containing progesterone and both progestins and estrogens are being tested. Some experts estimate that these other rings may be available in the early 1990s. The progesterone ring could be very useful for breastfeeding women, because it would not affect breast milk.

Transdermal patches constitute another delivery system that could provide slow, consistent release of contraceptive steroids to the bloodstream through the skin. Now being used to provide estrogen-replacement therapy to menopausal women, the transdermal patches can be worn on the body and replaced by the user as needed (ALZA Corporation, 1988b). In one system, three patches (each effective for seven days) would be worn consecutively for three weeks, followed by a week during which no patch or a placebo patch would be worn to allow menstrual bleeding to occur. Early clinical trials of this system were completed in 1988 and studies on improved patches were scheduled to begin in the United States in 1989.

The technology of *osmotic pills* could also be used for controlled release of contraceptive steroids. Osmotic pills allow for a gradual release of a drug encased in a semipermeable membrane. Because the drug is released continuously at controlled rates, lower and less frequent dosages are possible, thereby reducing the potential adverse effects associated with oral formulations that are absorbed quickly (ALZA Corporation, 1988a).

Many researchers believe that, in the long term, a *vaccine* could be the ideal contraceptive because it could be highly effective, long-acting, and eventually reversible. Three types of vaccines are currently being studied. One would immunize a woman against human chorionic gonadotrophin (hCG), a placental hormone that is needed in early pregnancy; the second would immunize against the hormone in the zona pellucida of the egg; and the third would work against the sperm (Harper, 1983a). Following an initial series of injections to establish immunity, a woman would need a periodic (probably annual) booster shot to prevent the return of fertility. Research on vaccines is at an early stage, and there are many technical problems to overcome. Nonetheless, it is possible that at least one version of the hCG antipregnancy vaccine could become available for use in some countries around the turn of the century (Segal, 1989). In 1988 the FDA approved the initiation of clinical research on a contraceptive vaccine in the United States.

One alternative to the contraceptive methods based on analogues of estrogen and progesterone is the use of *luteinizing hormone-releasing hormone (LHRH) analogues*, which control reproduction by affecting the pituitary gland (Schally et al., 1971; Guillemin et al., 1971). In early clinical trials, LHRH analogues have been effective in suppressing ovulation, and ovulation returned quickly once the drug was discontinued (Harper, 1983). It was originally thought that LHRH analogues could be administered by injection or nasal sprays; other possible modes of administration include suppository, cheek insert, or oral capsule (OTA, 1981). Researchers believed that LHRH analogues might have fewer side effects than combined oral contraceptives. However, clinical work has revealed many difficulties. LHRH analogues also block production of estrogen and progesterone in the ovaries; if these hormones are replaced by drug therapy, the resulting side effects might negate any advantages LHRH analogues have over existing steroidal methods (Wiedhaup, 1988).

Male Methods

Although sperm antigens have been tested for use in women, their use in a reversible vaccine for men is not considered feasible because destroying sperm production capability would lead to permanent sterility (Harper and Sanford, 1980). Animal studies using sperm antigens found an increase in tumors in male mice and more atherosclerosis in male monkeys (Alexander and Anderson, 1985). Because so much more research is needed to develop and test suitable antigens for a male vaccine, a male vaccine—reversible or permanent—will not be available for general use in this century.

Inhibin, a peptide derived from the testis, is thought to regulate production of follicle-stimulating hormone (FSH). More research is needed to understand the biology and to develop the specific form of inhibin needed for sperm suppression and to develop a specific regimen for its use. Nevertheless, animal studies suggest that an FSH-inhibiting drug might be effective without changing libido or potency.

Scientists are also studying ways to interfere with the fertilizing capacity of sperm as they mature while passing through the epididymis. In the 1960s, *gossypol*, a derivative of cotton seed, was found to cause male infertility in China. Although the rigor and documentation of many Chinese studies of gossypol are uncertain, the antifertility action of gossypol has been studied extensively and its effectiveness has been clearly demonstrated. Two major side effects threaten its potential usefulness: it can deprive the body of potassium (needed for normal muscle function), and its antifertility effect appears to be irreversible in some cases. Reduced sperm count can take two to three months to achieve, and the return of fertility may take at least three to four months (Harper, 1983). To date, no clinical studies of gossypol have been initiated in the United States. However, the principles underlying research on gossypol should enable scientists to explore other important areas in search of a nonhormonal, nonendocrine contraceptive method.

Modifications of Existing Methods

Significant *modifications of oral contraceptive formulations* have recently been introduced in Europe. Three new compounds—desogestrel, gestodene, and norgestimate—allow significant reductions in dosage compared with oral contraceptives currently on the market in the United States (Wiedhaup, 1988). A new oral contraceptive containing gestodene, for example, contains only about one hundredth the amount of contraceptive steroid contained in the first oral contraceptive marketed in the United States in the early 1960s (Segal, 1989). If the European manufacturers file for FDA approval, these new oral contraceptives may become available in the United States in the 1990s.

The main focus of research on natural family planning methods has been *devices for predicting ovulation* or detecting when ovulation has occurred in order to pinpoint more accurately the time for periodic abstinence. In some Western countries, the first models of a "personal rhythm clock," which uses a high-precision thermometer and calculator to interpret daily fluctuations in body temperature, and an "ovutimer," which analyzes changes in cervical mucus, are on the market.

Practical biochemical methods for prediction of ovulation, and therefore for improvements in natural family planning, can also be anticipated in the 1990s. Research on new *monoclonal antibodies*, which can be used to detect hormones produced by the ovary, is far advanced. Reliable detectors for ovulation based on urinalysis are already on the market. Research is also under way on ovarian markers of follicular growth and urinary estrogen assays to monitor follicular development (Institute for International Studies in Natural Family Planning, 1988). Research has also been carried out on the use of salivary electrolytes and glucose as an indicator of the fertile period (WHO, 1988).

New *hormone-releasing IUDs* and *modifications to copper IUDs* have recently been developed and tested (Sivin and Tatum, 1981; Luukkainen et al., 1987). A long-lasting copper IUD, which has a pregnancy rate of less than 1 percent, was introduced in the United States in June 1988. These methods provide highly effective long-term protection at relatively low cost with little risk for most women.

The search for new *spermicides*, especially those with virucidal properties, has taken on new importance as a consequence of the dramatic increase in sexually transmitted diseases. Several researchers are trying to develop new spermicides. Preliminary studies have found that propranolol, a *beta blocking agent* widely used in the treatment of cardiovascular disease, is an effective spermicide. One study involving 198 volunteers found a pregnancy rate of 3.9 pregnancies per 100 woman-years of use (Sherris, 1984). However, more work needs to be done on formulation and on research to increase effectiveness.

Disposable diaphragms containing spermicide have been developed but are not being vigorously pursued. One disposable diaphragm manufactured by G.D. Searle and Co. was approved by the FDA in the late 1970s but was withdrawn in 1980 when test marketing sales were low (Sherris, 1984). The FDA refused G.D. Searle's request for approval to market the product for sale without a prescription. GynoPharma is currently evaluating a new vaginal barrier very similar to the disposable diaphragm.

A *female condom*, developed in Europe in the early 1980s, is being tested in both Europe and the United States. Made of polyethylene plastic, the female condom consists of two flexible rings and a loose-fitting sheath that lines the vagina so that sperm cannot enter the cervix (International Planned Parenthood Federation, 1988). The larger ring at the open end secures the device outside the vagina, while a smaller ring at the closed end is inserted into the vagina and placed at the cervix. It is larger than a male condom, its use is controlled by the female, and the method may provide greater protection against sexually transmitted diseases.

Recently the FDA Medical Device Center allowed the marketing of two condoms: the "minicondom," a shorter version of a condom using adhesives (in 1988), and the "panty condom," a condom constructed so that it can be worn by the woman (in 1987). Because these products were considered to be substantially equivalent to products already on the market, no clinical studies of efficacy and safety had been required for FDA approval. In 1989 the status of both products changed: before the minicondom can be marketed, pregnancy rates must be included in the package labeling; and clearance for the panty condom was rescinded pending FDA reevaluation because of a change in the product's design.

Considerable work is also under way to develop a new type of *male condom* that substitutes synthetic materials such as silicone and polyurethane for latex. These materials could provide greater strength, uniformity, and durability and increased sensitivity compared with latex products.

Another research lead involves sterilization procedures. Current female sterilization procedures can be reversed only through use of complex microsurgery, which is expensive and not always successful. Researchers have been exploring various techniques for *reversible female sterilization*, but there are no major leads on the horizon. Clips, bands, fimbrial hoods, and plugs to obstruct the fallopian tubes have been tested, but none has proven to significantly increase reversibility.

Research on *transcervical sterilization*—the placement of various chemicals into the uterus at the opening of the oviduct—has been under way for 20 years. Such procedures would eliminate the risks associated with surgery, but none of them has proven very practical. Among the chemicals that have reached the stage of clinical trials are silver nitrate, quinacrine, phenol, ethanol-formaldehyde, and methylcyanoacrylate (Harper, 1983). Most of these chemicals cause scarring, which blocks the fallopian tubes. Researchers have also injected liquid silicone rubber into the fallopian tubes to form a barrier when it hardens. The main problems with sclerosing agents have been the high failure rates and the need for repeated installations. These techniques could also pose a greater risk of ectopic or tubal pregnancy. Reversibility is another concern, although the rubber plugs may prove to be removable (Harper, 1983).

In recent years, much research has been done on *reversible methods of male sterilization* and nonsurgical techniques to make the procedure easier and less expensive. Various valves and plugs that are inserted into the vas deferens to block sperm transport have been tested, but it has proven difficult to anchor them in the vas, and there have been problems with vas erosion and inflammatory reactions (Harper, 1983). The "Shug" device, which consists of two silicone plugs joined by a nylon thread, is in clinical trials in the United States. Early results are promising, but even if research continues to progress smoothly, it will be several years before the device could be approved and available (Program for Applied Research on Fertility Regulation, 1987; Contraceptive Research and Development Program, 1988).

Nonsurgical male sterilization techniques have involved the *injection of chemicals*, including methylcyanoacrylate, ethanol, and formaldehyde into the vas deferens. A great deal of additional research is needed to assess the efficacy and safety of these methods (Harper, 1983). In China, a sterilization technique in which a sclerosing chemical is injected into the vas deferens has been performed on over 1 million men (Segal, 1989). Another procedure uses the "no-scalpel" vasectomy technique developed in China, in which a small puncture rather than an incision is made in the scrotum to locate the vas.

METHODS AVAILABLE OUTSIDE THE UNITED STATES

Couples in Western Europe and in some less developed countries have a wider choice of contraceptive methods and greater access to the latest contraceptive technology than couples in the United States. In some European countries, contraceptive implants, new oral contraceptives, injectable contraceptives, and a variety of IUDs and sterilization devices that are not available in the United States are approved and marketed. These methods have been found to be safe and effective means of contraception.

Depo-Provera (depot-medroxyprogesterone acetate or DMPA), taken by injection every three months, has a failure rate of less than 1 pregnancy per 100 women per year. It was developed in the United States and is manufactured by the Upjohn Company in Europe. Depo-Provera has been given limited or general approval in about 90 countries, including Canada, Sweden, and the United Kingdom. An estimated 4 million women worldwide use Depo-Provera (Liskin and Blackburn, 1987). In 1978, after nearly four years of review, FDA declined to approve Depo-Provera for use as a contraceptive in the United States (see Chapter 7).

A two-month injectable, *Noristerat* (norethisterone enanthate or NET-EN), is manufactured by Schering AG in West Germany and is approved in more than 40 countries. Its failure rate is higher than Depo-Provera—about 2 pregnancies per 100 women per year. An estimated 800,000 women worldwide use Noristerat (Liskin and Blackburn, 1987). Both Mexico and China manufacture their own one-month injectables. It is estimated that there are over 300,000 users of injectables in Mexico and and over 1 million in China (Liskin and Blackburn, 1987). There are currently eight different injectable contraceptive compounds being marketed around the world (Kleinman, 1988).

NORPLANT® is a progestin-releasing contraceptive implant that is placed under the skin on the inside of a woman's upper arm. The implant, which is manufactured in Finland by Leiras Pharmaceuticals, can provide contraceptive protection for up to five years. The nonbiodegradable capsules containing levonorgestrel are inserted through a small incision and can be removed by a trained person when a pregnancy is desired, when their effectiveness declines, or if the user is troubled by side effects. A six-capsule version of NORPLANT® has been tested on more than 55,000 women in 31 countries and has been approved in at least 12 countries, including Finland in 1983 and Sweden in 1984 (Population Council, 1988). In August 1988, a New Drug Application was filled for NORPLANT® with the FDA. In April 1989 the Fertility and Maternal Health Drug Advisory Committee of the FDA unanimously recommended that NORPLANT® be approved for marketing in the United States. Wyeth has expressed interest in marketing NORPLANT®, if it is approved.

A newer version containing two rods (NORPLANT®-2) and providing contraceptive protection for up to three years has been approved in Finland; clinical trials are under way in nine other countries. Evaluation of NORPLANT®-2 has been delayed, however, because of problems with the supply of the polymer used to form the core of the two rods. Other versions of contraceptive implants using one rod are also undergoing clinical trials (Wiedhaup, 1988).

The main advantages of NORPLANT® are its high effectiveness (less than 1 pregnancy per 100 women per year), reversibility, and convenience; in addition, because NORPLANT® provides among the lowest levels of steroids of any steroidal method, it has a low incidence of serious adverse health consequences. Its disadvantages are that it must be inserted and removed by health professionals. In addition, it typically changes menstrual bleeding patterns, and the capsule's rods may be visible under the skin.

The *Multiload IUD*, which is used by a large proportion of all IUD users in Europe, has never been introduced into the United States. According to the manufacturer, Organon International, they consider the costs of liability insurance and of defending possible liability claims in the United States to be too high, and the negative publicity resulting from such claims to be potentially detrimental to sales in other countries (Wiedhaup, 1988). A variety of other IUDs are used in China and a few other countries, but they are not likely to be introduced to the American market.

For more than a decade, researchers have tested various chemicals that could be used to bring on a delayed menstrual period. The most advanced antiprogesterone, *RU-486*, currently thought to be most effective when used with prostaglandin analogues, was developed in France by Roussel-Uclaf. During the past five years, RU-486 has been tested in 15 countries, including France, Sweden, and the United States (Halpern, 1987). It was approved for use in France and China in 1988. Known generally as mifepristone and marketed in France under the trade name, Mifegyne, RU-486 is an antiprogesterone steroid that blocks the cells in the uterus from receiving progesterone, which is needed to support the fertilized egg. (RU-486 is discussed further in Chapter 4.)

The *Filshie clip*, made of titanium lined with silicone rubber, is a method of occluding the fallopian tubes during female sterilization. It has a low failure rate and is thought to cause less damage to the tubes, an important consideration should the woman request a reversal. The Filshie clip has been tested among more than 10,000 women worldwide and is approved for use in the United Kingdom and Canada (Liskin and Rinehart, 1985). *Ovablock* silicone plugs, used for female sterilization and thought to increase the prospects of reversibility, are already available in the Netherlands.

CONCLUSION

People in the United States currently have limited options for fertility control and fewer contraceptive choices than people in several other industrialized countries and in some developing countries as well. Some improvements in existing methods will be made in the next decade, and some highly effective new methods may become available in other countries. Some of these new methods will probably be safer, easier to use, less expensive, and more acceptable than existing methods. Other new methods will meet the needs of special population subgroups, such as lactating women or women over 35.

The prospects for having one or more fundamentally new methods available in the United States by the year 2000 are negligible. Contraceptive methods that are fundamentally different from existing technology, such as a contraceptive vaccine, are likely to have a greater positive impact on the consumer and society as a whole but will take considerable time to develop.

Some promising new methods, such as the contraceptive vaccine, for which much of the basic research has been completed, are not being developed at a rate that scientific knowledge would allow. Other methods have been approved by one or more European countries, but additional clinical trials in the United States are needed to qualify for FDA approval. Moreover, there are continuing opportunities for basic research in reproductive biology, which may yield significant contraceptive leads.

Accelerated efforts to develop and introduce new contraceptive products to the market would lead to a wider variety of contraceptive options for women and men in the United States and abroad and would result in safer, more effective, and more acceptable contraception for a much broader population than is being served by existing methods.

4

Values and
Contraceptive Development

The contraceptive development process cannot be adequately understood by focusing only on the potential gain in effectiveness or safety of a new method or on the profits a manufacturer projects for a new product. It is also important to understand the attitudes and values that influence the perception of individuals and groups regarding contraceptive practice and the need for new methods, as well as their desire for certain levels of risk, convenience, and cost and their willingness to support efforts to develop new contraceptives.

This chapter provides a sketch of some of the many facets of American values related to contraception and human reproduction. Although the committee did not attempt a comprehensive treatment, these issues are important and merit attention. One reason that we have not provided more detail is that the information needed for complete analysis of the history and sociology of American attitudes toward the control of human reproduction and their likely impact on contraceptive development is not available. Although there is a sizable scientific literature examining knowledge about, attitudes toward, and the practice of contraception, almost no research has been done on public opinion regarding contraceptive development. Thus, we cannot present a full-blown examination of this complex topic. Despite the shortcomings in available information, it is important to illustrate the range of attitudes and values related to contraceptive development that exist in the United States and to discuss the value conflicts that almost certainly have affected the development of new contraceptives. These conflicts, and the differences in attitudes on which they are based, are part of the full range of factors that influence contraceptive development in the United States.

41

ROOTS OF AMERICAN VALUES ON CONTRACEPTION

In comparison with some cultures, American attitudes toward reproduction and contraceptive use appear remarkably conservative; compared with other societies, we seem permissive and sexually liberated. Moreover, when examining the likely effects of values, attitudes, and beliefs on contraceptive development, it is not clear whose values are most decisive—those of pharmaceutical industry executives, those of the likely users of a new method, those of militant opponents of a potential new method, or those of some larger and less-well-defined public. It is also not clear how to evaluate the importance of the historical context in which these attitudes exist. Positive public attitudes may have encouraged support for contraceptive research and development at one time, but these attitudes may have changed partly in response to other changes, such as the legalization of abortion or the advent of AIDS, and interest in new methods may have increased or decreased.

Historical Perspectives

The history of fertility control has been marked by occasional efforts to promote contraceptive use as a means of ensuring a certain numerical balance or even the superiority of a particular group. Before World War II, for example, there was a concern about maintaining racial homogeneity in the United States, a factor that influenced some of those who promoted family planning and who drafted America's immigration laws (Reed, 1978). Some leaders in the black community have worried about what they termed the *genocide* inherent in white promotion and black acceptance of federally subsidized family planning services (Littlewood, 1977). Given the links between the eugenics movement and the birth control movement, it is not surprising that some in the black community have argued that government-supported, organized family planning programs were racist. In the 1960s, considerable controversy erupted when family planning centers were located in black communities, because some people thought these programs were designed specifically for minority communities (Joffe, 1986). Indeed, there is evidence that family planning clinics in small counties in the South were located in black areas, regardless of other measures of the need for such services (Billy, 1979). Despite the suspicion with which family planning was regarded in minority communities, minority women have used family planning services to meet their individual desires to prevent pregnancies and births. But there are people who feel uneasy about government support for fertility control and for contraceptive development. Moreover, for some Americans there is the added influence of deeply held cultural or religious values that cause them to question the appropriateness of efforts to influence reproductive choices or to help people control fertility.

While hostility to contraception exists in the United States, recent decades have witnessed a growing acceptance of the idea that fertility should be controlled and substantial increases in contraceptive practice to enhance individual and social welfare. Only modest differences exist in rates of practice among various economic, religious, and racial groups. Opposition to family planning appears to be limited to a tiny minority of Americans, almost all of whom oppose abortion, sterilization, or modern methods of contraception for religious reasons. Despite the widespread practice of modern contraception and the overall favorable attitudes toward fertility control, there is no broad public demand for the development of new contraceptives. Resistance to the notion of separating sex from reproduction, which may have slowed the development of some contraceptives in the past (Potts, 1988), has been replaced with concern about the safety and appropriateness of different means of fertility control as a principal attitudinal barrier to development efforts. Changing attitudes toward sex, women, work, and the family have become increasingly important determinants of the nation's orientation toward fertility control, and these attitudes may now be more favorable to contraceptive development than in the past. If the economic importance of women in the work force continues to increase and is expressed in terms of greater political activity, their preferences for particular contraceptive products may become a more important factor in contraceptive development efforts and public pressure for new products.

Religious Perspectives

Current American attitudes toward contraception and human reproduction are often rooted in beliefs and values molded by the nation's dominant religious traditions. It is useful to briefly note the highlights of what those traditions have had to say about contraceptive practice. Although the desire to control fertility and the existence of contraceptive devices date to primitive times (Noonan, 1965), contraceptive use has often been a controversial practice for believers of all sorts. The societal disapproval that was manifested in religious prohibitions has often been incorporated into secular law. Both the religious and secular restrictions were, in turn, influenced by society's attitudes toward the role of women, marriage, and the family (Gordon, 1976).

In the Orthodox Jewish tradition, sexuality is considered a natural function of human beings that satisfies values other than procreation (Bleich, 1981). But, although it is viewed as a natural function, sexuality was historically not permitted unfettered expression, because "[r]ecognition and sanctification of the multiple values inherent in the sexual act do not bestow the right to thwart its procreative role" (Bleich, 1981:55). Orthodox tradition does not permit contraceptive use unless "pregnancy represents a health hazard to the mother or child, or when previous children have been born defective" (Kertzer, 1978:58). In contrast, Reform and Conservative Judaism have supported a more liberal position on contraceptive practice. The Central Conference of American Rabbis (Reform) approved the use of contraceptives for economic, social, and health reasons in

1930 and were joined in this position in 1935 by the Conservative Rabbinical Assembly (Kertzer, 1978). The Orthodox tradition appears to have little influence on the contraceptive behavior of most American Jews or on their support for the development of new contraceptive technology. Sample surveys consistently find Jews to be among the most liberal group in the United States with respect to attitudes toward contraception and abortion (Jacqueline D. Forrest, unpublished tabulations of the 1982 National Survey of Family Growth).

Like its contemporary Roman counterpart, the early Christian church was generally opposed to contraception. It valued an ascetic ideal that favored celibacy. Later, the church was much influenced by the Stoics and others who believed that legitimate sexual activity was distinguished by its procreative purpose (Noonan, 1965). This view was strongly reinforced by Saint Augustine, who also found the value of marriage in its procreative purpose. Thus, efforts to frustrate procreation by contraception were generally condemned.

The Roman Catholic church has in general continued to adhere to these early Christian traditions. Although the church sanctioned intercourse for married couples for whom reproduction was not possible, its teaching consistently asserted the goodness of procreation and remained opposed to contraception. In 1930, Pope Pius XI's encyclical *Casti Connubii* affirmed that the goal of marriage was procreation and condemned all contraceptive use except periodic abstinence or rhythm. Despite the fact that a papal commission appointed after Vatican II to review the church's position on family planning recommended that married couples be allowed to use contraceptives, in 1968 Pope Paul VI reaffirmed the church's disapproval of what Catholics refer to as artificial birth control (Murphy, 1981). The Catholic church's formal opposition to any method of contraception except periodic abstinence has remained unchanged over the last two decades.

The Catholic church's prohibition of all contraceptives but periodic abstinence (or the rhythm method) has not generally been observed by Catholics in the United States. Overall levels of contraceptive practice are very similar among Catholics and non-Catholics in the United States (Goldscheider and Mosher, 1988). There is no reason to think that Catholics in general would be more opposed to the development of new methods than members of other religious groups.

Protestant churches were generally in agreement with the Catholic church in opposing birth control until 1930. During that year, the Lambeth Conference of the Church of England recognized abstinence and permitted the use of contraceptives when abstinence was not possible. In 1931 the Committee on Marriage and Home of the Federal Council of Churches in the United States also permitted the use of contraceptives in some circumstances. Their position has been generally followed by all Protestant churches in the United States with the exception of the Lutheran church and certain fundamentalist churches (Murphy, 1981). With few exceptions, most Protestant denominations now permit contraceptive use, at least in some circumstances, and there are no data to suggest that American Protestantism is a significant impediment to faster contraceptive development.

While these religious traditions may not significantly influence individual contraceptive practice, they may play a role in people's willingness to publicly support contraceptive development. Contraceptive use is largely a private matter, and private behavior may diverge from publicly held positions. People shaped by certain religious traditions or living in communities influenced by those traditions may be reluctant to advocate openly and strongly the development of better means of preventing births, even if they are using contraception themselves. The climate of hostility created by certain religiously motivated opponents of different contraceptive methods is cited by some people as an element in pharmaceutical industry decisions not to support contraceptive development, but it is impossible to establish how important such opposition has really been.

Legal Perspectives

The impact of religion on contraceptive practice and attitudes toward the development of new methods may be difficult to specify, but the importance of the American legal system is clear and, like other aspects of the society, it too was influenced by the religious orientations of Americans. By the nineteenth century, laws began to regulate contraceptive use in the United States. Early attempts by the state to control contraceptive use took the form of restricting distribution of products or information about them by equating such information with obscenity. The primary example of this strategy was the Comstock Act, a federal statute enacted in 1873, which prohibited the mailing of "obscene or crime-inciting matter." Passage of this statute and the many state statutes that were modeled on it was rooted in religious objections to contraception. In addition to popular moral and ideologically based opposition to contraception, some people believed that the increasing use of contraceptives would contribute to a decline in the birth rate, which was already well under way in the nineteenth century but which still worried those who associated rapid population growth with American prosperity (Degler, 1980).

The first significant break in the legal prohibition of contraceptive use came in 1936, when a federal court of appeals ruled that the Comstock Act did not prohibit the distribution of contraceptives by physicians. However, state statutes modeled on the Comstock Act were not affected by the decision. Although access to contraception increased, especially for those able to pay for services from a physician, it was not until 1965 in *Griswold v. Connecticut* (431 U.S. 687 [1965]) that a state statute modeled after the federal Comstock Act was successfully challenged. Although the justices in *Griswold* differed in their rationale for striking down the statute, the case is regarded as a landmark in the establishment of a constitutionally protected right to privacy, which has continued to be especially significant in reproductive rights cases. Subsequent cases have further established the importance of autonomy and choice in the area of contraceptive use.

Read in light of subsequent cases, the teaching of *Griswold* is that the Constitution protects individual decisions in matters of childbearing from unjustified intrusion by the state. Although the Constitution protects the rights of individuals to have access to contraceptives, legal controversy remains. The extent to which parents have a legal role in reproductive decisions by their minor children and the extent to which religiously affiliated institutions involved in family planning activities may be supported by the federal government have been especially controversial.

CONTEMPORARY VALUE CONFLICTS: STERILIZATION AND ABORTION

No other aspects of contraceptive development and use have been as controversial, or as hotly debated by those with different religious and legal orientations, as sterilization and abortion. Americans' attitudes and values about these methods of fertility control highlight the problems that development of new methods poses for some people. Historically, concern about preventing births focused on contraception because, although sterilization and abortion were practiced, it was not until the early twentieth century that medically safe means of sterilization and abortion were developed (Mohr, 1978). Once safe procedures became available, these methods were used with greater frequency. For very different reasons, they became more controversial than other means of controlling fertility.

The early association of sterilization with the eugenics movement largely accounts for persistent mistrust among some populations toward those who advocate its use (Reed, 1978). Indiana enacted the first state law authorizing mandatory sterilization of certain persons in 1907. It is estimated that 70,000 persons have been compulsorily sterilized in Indiana and other states since then. As of 1985, 17 states had legislation authorizing sterilization of certain persons (Areen, 1985). One such statute was reviewed by the Supreme Court in *Buck v. Bell* (274 U.S. 200 [1927]). In an opinion written by Justice Oliver Wendell Holmes, Jr., the Court upheld the constitutionality of a Virginia law that permitted mandatory sterilization of "mental defectives." Justice Holmes reasoned:

> It is better for all the world, if instead of waiting to execute degenerate offspring for crime, or to let them starve for their imbecility, society can prevent those who are manifestly unfit from continuing their kind. The principle that sustained compulsory vaccination is broad enough to cover cutting the Fallopian tubes. Three generations of imbeciles are enough.

The Supreme Court has never overruled *Buck*, although its significance has been undermined by subsequent decisions such as *Skinner v. Oklahoma* (316 U.S.

365 [1942]), in which the Supreme Court held that Jack Skinner, a convicted criminal, was not required to undergo mandatory sterilization as provided by Oklahoma law. The law, which was concerned with the inheritability of criminal tendencies, allowed for the imprisonment and sterilization of any person convicted of a felony more than twice.

Abuses associated with sterilization have not been confined to actions of states in connection with the mentally disabled or criminals. In 1973 it was learned that federal funds had been used in Alabama to sterilize the Relf sisters, black minors ages 12 and 14, without their consent or the consent of their parents (Areen, 1985). As a result of successful litigation, federal regulations were changed and now provide that federal funds cannot be used to sterilize minors under 21 or mentally incompetent persons. Despite the fact that male and female sterilization together constitutes the most widely used method of fertility control among married couples in the United States, and despite the fact that many courts have tightened the standards that must be met before a retarded child or adult can be sterilized, in minority communities particularly, the abuses associated with sterilization have helped foster distrust of many promoters of contraceptive services, even though there has been no apparent impact on the levels of contraceptive practice, including sterilization (Weisbord, 1975).

Changing technology has also influenced the public's view of different contraceptive options. The development of highly effective long-term methods may also help to narrow the perceived difference between sterilization and other forms of contraception. Today it is possible to reverse surgical sterilization, although the procedures for doing so are complex and expensive and have a relatively low success rate. Highly effective long-term methods of contraception, such as NORPLANT®, are claimed by some to be, in effect, sterilization, although pregnancy rates among those discontinuing these methods to become pregnant are similar to those observed following discontinuation of other methods. Moreover, the highly effective long-term (but temporary) contraceptives currently under development may replace surgical sterilization as the preferred method of preventing births in certain populations, such as mentally disabled persons.

Without doubt, abortion is the most controversial method of preventing births. Because little was known about pregnancy or development of the fetus, no laws governed abortion in the United States until the late nineteenth century. American common law adhered to principles concerning the fetus inherited from English common law (Luker, 1984b). Abortion was not a crime prior to the point at which the women felt the fetus move and, even after this quickening, abortion was not considered the murder of a person. By the end of the nineteenth century, however, every state had passed legislation severely restricting abortion. It was not until the mid-twentieth century that widespread efforts to liberalize these restrictive laws began.

The movement toward less restrictive abortion laws reached its peak in the 1973 decision of the Supreme Court in *Roe v. Wade* (410 U.S. 113 [1973]). In

Roe, the Court declared unconstitutional a Texas abortion statute that prohibited abortion except to save the life of the mother. The Court reasoned that the right of privacy includes the decision of a woman whether to terminate her pregnancy. Under *Roe*, the woman's privacy right is not absolute, however; it is subject to state interests in maternal health and the potential life of the fetus. The interest in health becomes compelling at the end of the first trimester of pregnancy, and the interest in potential life becomes compelling at the point at which the fetus becomes viable. Even after viability, a woman can obtain an abortion in some circumstances because a state is able to legislate to protect the fetus and prohibit abortion only if an abortion were not necessary to preserve the life and health of the mother. In *Roe* the Court also declared that the fetus is not a person within the meaning of the Fourteenth Amendment, and it refused to decide the question of when life begins. The *Roe* decision has been affirmed in subsequent decisions (Glendon, 1987), but one recent decision (*Webster v. Reproductive Health Services*, 109 S. Ct. 3040 [1989]) suggests that far-reaching changes may occur, particularly with respect to state-mandated restrictions on access to abortion.

Although abortion remains a subject of enormous controversy in the United States, data from public opinion polls indicate that a substantial number of Americans, more than 85 percent in some surveys, approve of abortion in some circumstances; approval is highest when a women's health is in jeopardy (Rossi and Sitaraman, 1988). Furthermore, these attitudes have changed very little since the mid-1970s. Citing data from a variety of polls, Lamanna concludes (1984:4) that the data on people's attitudes toward abortion have a basic tripartite pattern that is consistent across researchers and time periods. Approximately 20 percent of Americans would forbid abortion under any circumstances except to save the mother's life. About 25 percent support the position as defined in *Roe v. Wade*. Everyone else is in between, approving of abortion in some circumstances, but not in others. In general, Lamanna observes, the American people support abortion for hard reasons, such as risk to a mother's life, risk to her physical health, the risk of a genetically defective child, and pregnancy resulting from rape or incest, but oppose it for soft reasons, such as being unmarried or a teenager, not being able to support a child, or simply not wanting a child.

Support for abortion also depends on when during pregnancy an abortion is performed (Glendon, 1987). Although public opinion polls suggest the presence of a broad middle group that might be characterized as reluctantly pro-choice, their numbers have not been felt in public debates and discussions of abortion; those who hold views at either end of the spectrum of opinion have set the tone for abortion discussions. The distaste many people feel toward abortion and the increased visibility of those who oppose it may have served as disincentives in the contraceptive development process.

Attitudes toward abortion do not exist in isolation. Attitudes toward abortion and contraception are often linked: some who are opposed to abortion also have attitudes about women, work, and the family that are threatened by the easy availability and widespread use of contraception to control childbearing. Studies undertaken by Luker (1984b) and Joffe (1986) underscore the fact that, because pro-life and pro-choice advocates disagree about a host of issues related to women, work, sex, and family, they are often at odds not only on the question of abortion, but also on the subject of contraception.

The controversy associated with abortion has spilled over recently into discussions of the morality of new fertility control methods, such as RU-486. This controversy may have become aggravated because scientific advances have blurred the clear distinctions that once were seen to mark the boundaries between stages of human development and, therefore, between contraception and abortion. The action of some new methods, such as RU-486, which can be used very early in pregnancy before implantation occurs, makes them particularly controversial and, therefore, has reduced the number of organizations and scientists willing to become involved in their development.

The Link Between Contraceptive Development and Abortion

In addition to the link between attitudes about abortion and contraception, there is another interface between contraceptive development and abortion. Often women seeking abortion have experienced a contraceptive failure or have discontinued contraception because of perceived risks or unacceptable side effects or because they were in the process of considering other contraceptive options, including sterilization. The high prevalence of sterilization in the United States is due in part to the experience of contraceptive failure and in part to the limited acceptability and often low effectiveness of other contraceptive options available to older women. Studies in less developed countries suggest that similar relationships exist among contraceptive development, the demand for sterilization, and abortion, although in many countries the lack of safe abortion services or of easy access to a range of contraceptive choices compounds people's problems.

The extent to which abortion is available may also affect a woman's choice and use of contraception. If abortion is safe, legal and readily available, a woman might choose a safer but less effective contraceptive method. Conversely, if abortion is not readily available, a woman might select a more efficacious but also riskier contraceptive. The interdependence between abortion and contraception is such that the development of a safe and highly effective contraceptive could significantly reduce the frequency of abortion. One recent study indicates that as many as half of all unintended pregnancies resulting in abortion were the result of contraceptive failure (Henshaw and Silverman, 1988).

The link between contraception and abortion is also important because the mechanisms of action of different contraceptives have, in the minds of some people, clouded the differences between contraception and abortion. For those who believe that life begins at the moment of conception, any method that acts after that point is unacceptable. Although this is a metaphysical and religious issue and not a scientific one, it is worth noting that most scientists think conception is best represented as a process and the precise points at which it is initiated and at which it is completed are matters of definition. It is difficult to maintain that fertilization per se can produce a unique genetic identity or individual. The phenomenon of identical twinning, for example, may occur several days after fertilization. Implantation does not occur until the sixth or seventh postfertilization day, when there is contact with the bed of the uterus (endometrium) and further exchange thereafter between the mother and the recently formed conceptus.

Prevention of pregnancy during the interval between fertilization and onset of the first menstrual period, euphemistically referred to as *interception*, raises a new array of medical and ethical concerns. For many people, the critical point in human development is implantation rather than fertilization. In this view, implantation is crucial because it marks the point at which we know with empirical certainty that a new human entity with a unique genetic identity exists. Moreover, pregnancy cannot routinely be diagnosed before implantation. As a consequence, a woman cannot determine with certainty that she is pregnant until after implantation. Those who see implantation as the decisive stage believe that an intervention that acts during the period between fertilization and implantation resembles a contraceptive rather than an abortifacient because the interruption takes place before a pregnancy can be confirmed.

New technology used in the treatment of infertility has focused attention on the interval between fertilization and implantation, and a great deal of new information has been obtained recently from studies of in vitro fertilization (IVF). The Ethics Committee of the American Fertility Society refers to the first 14 days after conception as the "preembryonic stage" (American Fertility Society, 1986). It is generally agreed by those examining the ethical issues posed by IVF that, from the completion of normal fertilization, the conceptus is entitled to increased "respect," compared with other cells in the human body. Most nonreligious bodies, however, stop short of a firm definition as to when meaningful human life begins. Nevertheless, these developments serve to heighten the concern of those who oppose fertility control from the very earliest stages of fertilization that new methods of contraception could act after fertilization. This, coupled with the interdiction of some religious groups against almost all forms of modern contraception, provides a continuous source of potential conflict and controversy, the net result of which is probably to discourage both public and private investment in new contraceptive development.

RU-486

A new generation of compounds has recently appeared that are capable of interfering with the production of progesterone, the hormone essential for pregnancy. Two of these have been shown to be effective abortifacients (Nieman et al., 1987; Crooij et al., 1988). Other agents, which have been introduced for purposes unrelated to contraception, also cause early pregnancy loss. The potentially most important of these compounds from the contraceptive point of view is RU-486. When RU-486 is used in combination with prostaglandins (agents that cause uterine contractions), pregnancy termination before the 45th day of pregnancy is successful in 95 percent of the cases (Ulmann and DuBois, 1986). Use of RU-486 would reduce the need for surgical termination of pregnancy.

The publicity surrounding RU-486 has focused renewed attention on the ways that different contraceptives work. For some, RU-486 is entirely acceptable. For others, it is potentially acceptable if it is used before there is recognized evidence of pregnancy in the form of a missed menstrual period. For still others, the fact that RU-486 might act after the completion of the fertilization process makes it completely unacceptable.

Discussions of the ethical aspects of the development and use of RU-486 and similar agents are compounded by the fact that such drugs may also have potentially important noncontraceptive applications. Introduction of RU-486 for any purpose in the United States probably would be difficult because of widespread concern among medical scientists and pharmaceutical company executives about a conservative backlash against them, including the risk of economic boycott of manufacturers and distributors. A lack of strong public support has added to this climate of uncertainty and has resulted in a lack of research in the United States on RU-486 and other methods that, in some cases, are in their final stages of development abroad.

WOMEN'S PERSPECTIVES ON REPRODUCTION AND SOCIAL ROLES

Women have an obvious interest in controlling fertility because only they can become pregnant and give birth. Women must be concerned with the timing and spacing of births and, indeed, the decision to have children in ways that men may avoid. Women are more affected by pregnancy and childrearing than men and, as a consequence, their ability to pursue different options in life are often sharply circumscribed. To the extent that women can control reproduction, and thereby increase their ability to engage in activities unrelated to childbearing, they can move to equalize responsibilities with men for home and children (Petchesky, 1984).

The interrelationship between the perceived social benefits of a certain demographic balance and women's desire to control fertility has been particularly important in the twentieth century. Concern about the falling birth rate and the trend toward smaller families in the United States, evident in the beginning of the century, caused Theodore Roosevelt to brand women who avoided having children as "criminal[s] against the race . . . the object of contemptuous abhorrence by healthy people" (Gordon, 1976:136). Many people feared that members of the Yankee stock would be overwhelmed numerically—and hence politically—by immigrants, nonwhites, and the poor, all of whom had higher birth rates. Some people also viewed fertility control as a rebellion against women's primary duty of motherhood (Reed, 1978). Some women agreed with these concerns, but others objected either because they thought that fertility control was an issue of self-determination, or because they sought the expanded options for women that smaller families or childlessness might permit (Gordon, 1976).

The controversy generated by the low growth rates of native whites and by race suicide beliefs was brief—it was largely over by 1910—but its effects are important to an understanding of contemporary attitudes toward contraceptive development and use. The controversy freed some feminists to argue explicitly for contraception as a means of giving women freedom to control their lives. And the controversy exposed splits among women that have had enduring significance.

From 1942, when the Birth Control Federation of America changed its name to the Planned Parenthood Federation of America, to the 1960s, birth control was explicitly identified with the family. The success of this orientation helped to bring about the involvement of women in birth control issues in the 1960s. What was missing in the evolution of the birth control movement in the United States was an approach explicitly oriented to individual women's rights and health concerns. Despite the involvement of the medical profession in all aspects of contraceptive development and practice, many women felt that their health concerns were ignored or at least downplayed.

The medical orientation of most contraceptive services has reinforced the view among some women that adequate account has not been taken of their social and economic concerns. In the United States today, women generally receive contraceptives from private physicians or medically oriented family planning clinics. Although almost all family planning specialists argue that the ideal method of contraception would be one that would be safely available over the counter and without the need for any medical supervision, most currently available modern methods involve some risk and therefore require varying degrees of medical supervision. Thus, for example, pelvic examinations are needed prior to the insertion of an IUD or the fitting of a diaphragm. Proper utilization of the pill is dependent on knowledge and understanding of a woman's medical history.

An expanded understanding of the factors that should be taken into account in contraceptive development—what is being called "the user perspective" (Bruce, 1987)—would involve considerations well beyond a narrow focus on technical efficacy. From the standpoint of a woman seeking to avoid pregnancy, it is the method that fails when she errs in its use, when the method is flawed or too expensive, or when its risks, side effects, mode of administration, or use make it unacceptable to her or her partner. In short, a method fails because it does not meet a woman's basic needs, which include the need to maintain her health, lifestyle, and well-being and perhaps the need to keep her options open about future childbearing (Petchesky, 1984).

Many women who want to control their fertility desire to do so in a context that permits sharing the responsibility with men. Thus, they support the development of male contraceptives because they wish to equalize the burden of contraceptive practice. At the same time, however, there is appreciation that for many women reliance on men to prevent birth is not feasible (Petchesky, 1984).

The 1960s and 1970s saw the emergence of birth control as a key concern of the women's movement. Yet the involvement of the women's movement has not resulted in overwhelming support for the development of new contraceptives. In part this is the case because contemporary feminism has paid more attention to keeping abortion legal and accessible than to the development of new contraceptives. Moreover, the feminist health movement has often been critical of the family planning establishment and of specific contraceptives, including Depo-Provera, the IUD, and the pill (Joffe, 1986). This critique has often overshadowed concurrent feminist pleas for improved contraceptives. Even though there may be a common understanding that preventing births has special significance for women, their views are influenced by a variety of factors including race, religion, social class, education, and labor force participation. The women's movement has not subordinated this diversity to a single vision of what is best for women simply as women.

CONCLUSION

A large number of factors influence the nation's commitment to contraceptive development and the willingness of public and private organizations to invest in the field. The links between contraceptive development and abortion have enlarged the impact of groups opposing abortion on contraceptive research and development. These groups may influence a congressional decision to fund research or override industry's inclination to develop and market new contraceptive products.

Low fertility in Western industrialized nations, together with the perception that only women are affected, has contributed to the lack of public interest and political support for contraceptive development. The priority given to contraceptive development has been low because of more pressing demands for funding. Even the Planned Parenthood Federation and other family planning organizations have assigned contraceptive development a lower priority than other needs they perceive to be more immediate.

Despite religious opposition by some people and a history of minority group concerns about suspected abuses, recent decades have demonstrated a much greater demand in the United States for safe and effective contraceptive technology. These demands are based on a now-widespread view that the ability to regulate childbearing is a basic human right and is of primary importance to people's health and well-being. Nevertheless, the search for new and better contraceptives is hampered by a weak commitment to reproductive research and contraceptive development on the part of Congress, private foundations, and the pharmaceutical industry. Although millions of people may value the development of new contraceptives highly, these values have not influenced the federal government's contraceptive development program nor that of private industry. Given the importance of developing safer, more effective, more acceptable or more convenient contraceptives, it is surprising that the growing positive attitudes toward development have not been reflected in greater public support of policies and programs to enhance the likelihood that new methods will be developed.

In the 1960s and early 1970s, many women who might have supported the development of new contraceptive methods were concerned about the goals of those advocating government subsidized birth control, about the role and influence of the medical profession in contraceptive development and provision, and about the lack of concern for the users' perspective. Nonetheless, for all women, safer and more effective methods of preventing births, which take account of women's social and economic conditions and their changing life-styles, are critically important. Alliances among scientists, clinicians, and women are probably more possible today than at any time in the past. The likelihood that support for contraceptive development will increase may be dependent on whether these alliances can be formed and sustained.

5

Organizational Structure of Contraceptive Development

This chapter examines the roles played by the organizations involved in contraceptive development. We review the activities of government, universities, industry, and nonprofit organizations, evaluate how these groups interact, and discuss how organizational relationships affect contraceptive development. It is the sum of the actions of the full range of institutions in the contraceptive development field, together with the interdependencies of those actions, that determines the direction and pace of scientific research on new methods of contraception, the rate of new product development and marketing, and eventually the availability of contraceptive products throughout society.

This chapter concentrates on contraceptive development efforts in the United States. It is important to note, however, that contraceptive research and development in other countries have been noteworthy. European drug companies and scientists have made important contributions to the field, as has the contraceptive research of several institutions in the developing world such as the Indian Council of Medical Research and scientists working at medical schools in Chile and Mexico. The World Health Organization's Special Programme of Research, Development, and Research Training in Human Reproduction, established in 1972, has also undertaken significant research and development activities and has helped coordinate the worldwide effort to promote contraceptive development.

Organizations involved in basic research, product development, clinical testing, and marketing of contraceptives constitute a heterogeneous mix of institutional types. There is a private-enterprise sector, which includes both very large, multiproduct, multinational firms and a number of smaller firms with limited product lines. The large firms are vertically integrated, with major research divisions, manufacturing operations, and marketing and distribution systems. Smaller firms typically are less fully integrated, choosing to purchase more services from others. Considerations of profitability lead private-sector firms not to concentrate their research on advancing basic scientific knowledge, for advances at this level are not typically patentable. Rather, large firms tend to support applied research leading directly to saleable products.

The public sector has four important, although often uncoordinated, roles in contraceptive development. First, it is the major source of funding, primarily through the National Institutes of Health, for the basic research in human reproduction that the private sector finds unprofitable but that is carried out by universities and nonprofit organizations. That research has potential social value in expanding fundamental scientific knowledge. The government also carries out basic scientific research itself at the National Institutes of Health. In both of these capacities, the public sector provides the financial resources to support research activities that cannot be expected to be financed solely by the private sector.

From time to time the government takes on a second role in supporting activities usually left to the private sector. This is the case with contraceptive development for which the government provides direct support for product development through funding from the National Institutes of Health and the U.S. Agency for International Development. In this case, the government is responding to the perceived social need for additional contraceptive products and the fact that the private sector is not successfully undertaking the development work needed to produce those products.

The public sector performs a third role when it regulates the development of new contraceptives by means of the activities of the Food and Drug Administration (see Chapter 7) or, through the legal system, provides a means to adjudicate disputes about the adverse consequences of contraceptive use (see Chapter 8). Finally, the public sector also acts as a consumer when it purchases contraceptives for public programs in the United States (through the Department of Health and Human Services) and developing countries (through the Agency for International Development).

Nonprofit organizations constitute another component of the contraceptive development field. Nonprofit organizations consist of foundations, which provide funding for research, the training of scientists, and other purposes, and operating organizations, such as the Population Council, Family Health International, the Program for Appropriate Technology in Health (PATH), as well as universities and university-based programs such as the Contraceptive Research and Development Program (CONRAD) at Eastern Virginia Medical School. International organizations such as the World Health Organization and the World Bank are also active in the field. Similar to government, nonprofit and international organizations assist in financing activities that are unprofitable for private firms (though socially desirable) and in carrying out those activities. Such work involves activities from basic research through the distribution of contraceptive information and devices. Nonprofit organizations supplement the role of government agencies, while avoiding many of the political and other constraints government faces.

The organizational landscape of the contraceptive development field is shaped by attempts to deal with problems of funding, performing basic and applied research, and product development and marketing. Contraceptive innovation requires very sophisticated scientific research and product development and, as a consequence, is very expensive. Moreover, a significant proportion of consumers cannot afford all the costs involved in developing and supplying contraceptive products. Nevertheless, there are strong societal interests in broad access to contraceptives. Serving these societal interests involves some activities that bring clear, private benefits to consumers who have adequate ability to pay, similar benefits to other users whose ability to pay is extremely limited, and societal benefits (for example, from basic research and applied product development). This complex reward structure has resulted in different types of organizations becoming active in the field.

Each element in the organizational structure typically performs a distinct role. An organization's environment, particularly the incentive structure to which each type of organization responds, is as important as internal organizational characteristics in determining how, and how well, its role will be performed. Private firms, for example, can be expected to meet societal needs only when their expected financial rewards exceed all costs—including those associated with research, product development, meeting regulatory standards, incurring product liability losses, and so on. Anything that decreases profitability will reduce the role of the private sector. Anything that decreases profitability for large firms while increasing it for smaller firms will affect the size distribution of firms engaged in contraceptive-related activities. Likewise, whatever the motivation of the individuals' working there may be to serve social and humanitarian goals, nonprofit organizations, including universities, can be expected to be successful only insofar as they obtain funds from individuals, private foundations, or government. Anything that reduces or limits federal government and foundation support will lessen the involvement of the nonprofit organizations in contraceptive development activities.

A DIVERSITY OF EXPERTISE

The development and successful introduction of a new contraceptive require a wide variety of expertise—from a knowledge of the cutting edge of biomedical science to an ability to master and comply with complex regulatory requirements. Contraceptive development and introduction also require a pool of highly skilled personnel and a large amount of capital. To be successful, a large number of scientific, legal, financial, manufacturing, and marketing activities must be carried out and managed simultaneously.

Many organizational structures could accomplish the required tasks from basic research to postmarketing surveillance. In fact, a variety of organizations of different types, sizes, and complexity with a wide spectrum of personnel and missions have been involved in the development and marketing of new contraceptives. The kinds of organizations that have dominated different tasks have changed over time. Why large pharmaceutical companies, nonprofit organizations, government agencies, and intergovernmental bodies entered or left a particular arena frequently cannot be fully documented. But it is possible to sketch the organizational structure of the contraceptive development field over time and to assess its impact on the development of new technology.

Since the late 1960s the participation of the private sector in contraceptive development has diminished in the United States. The decline in private-sector involvement, as well as increases in funding from the National Institutes of Health and the Agency for International Development, has meant growth in the role of the public sector and of nonprofit organizations, including universities. Government funding for research in reproductive biology and contraceptive development increased substantially between 1973 and 1987, while investments in contraceptive-related research and development by major drug companies declined substantially, although the precise change is impossible to specify. As a result of these changing patterns of funding and research, a small number of private nonprofit organizations have become major forces in contraceptive development.

Only large pharmaceutical firms are capable of undertaking all aspects of the development and marketing of new methods on their own. Smaller organizations typically specialize in particular activities or stages of the development process. One group may be most involved with a particular type of research or with the development of a product concept for a new contraceptive method; another may fund research and development activities; others specialize in biological evaluation, engineering design, or toxicological or clinical testing; still others concentrate on clinical trials of new methods, application for regulatory approval, or the introduction of the new technology.

Just as a variety of organizations are involved in research and development efforts, so too are several different organizational types providing funding for the development of new methods. The Center for Population Research at the National Institute of Child Health and Human Development and the Office of Population at the Agency for International Development are the two major sources of federal government support for contraceptive development. The Rockefeller and Andrew W. Mellon foundations are the major foundations providing support for contraceptive research and development. The funding of contraceptive development is discussed in detail in Chapter 6.

In an appendix to this chapter, we list the organizations that are currently involved in contraceptive research and development in the United States. The appendix includes U.S. government agencies, private firms, foundations, nonprofit organizations, universities, and international organizations that are currently supporting contraceptive research and development activities. Because information on research and development activities and expenditures is proprietary and so many organizations do not release it, the appendix is not as complete as we would like. Nevertheless, the available data provide a clear sense of both the range of organizations active in the field and the range of potential products being studied.

In the sections that follow we describe the major types of organizations involved in contraceptive development. In addition to two federal agencies, NIH and AID, and one large pharmaceutical firm, Ortho Pharmaceutical Corp., more than a dozen private companies of different sizes, from very small to multimillion dollar, are conducting contraceptive development activities. Also actively trying to develop new contraceptive technology are nonprofit organizations. Three large European pharmaceutical firms and the Human Reproduction Programme of the World Health Organization are also involved in a range of contraceptive development activities. These organizations are working on products ranging from improved condoms to antipregnancy vaccines, including all the potential innovations described in Chapter 3.

The Pharmaceutical Industry

Over the past three decades, at least nine large U.S. pharmaceutical companies have been involved in research and development of new contraceptives. By the mid-1980s, however, only Ortho Pharmaceutical Corp. (a subsidiary of Johnson & Johnson) continued a significant contraceptive research and development program. In Europe, three companies, Organon International, Schering AG, and Roussel-Uclaf (a subsidiary of Hoechst Pharmaceuticals), have significant in-house contraceptive research and development programs. The U.S. companies that have for all practical purposes abandoned significant efforts on new contraceptive research include Syntex Laboratories, Inc.; G.D. Searle & Co.; Parke-Davis & Co.; Merck, Sharp & Dohme Co.; the Upjohn Company; Mead Johnson; Wyeth-Ayerst Laboratories; and Eli Lilly and Company (Djerassi, 1989, and personal communication to the committee). Whether any of these companies will resume research aimed at developing new contraceptives for the American market is uncertain, but it seems to be increasingly unlikely in the near future.

Companies must make difficult decisions about which areas of research are most likely to provide a satisfactory return on investment and ensure corporate growth. These decisions are affected by market trends, by the possibility of achieving significant advances leading to new patent-protected products meeting consumer needs, and by a company's history and place in the market. Managers must also take into account the often significant opportunity costs when selecting new products to develop. All the large pharmaceutical companies previously involved in contraceptive development have product lines in areas unrelated to fertility regulation. Research and development funds have increasingly been allocated to these other less controversial and potentially more profitable products.

The development of a new product entails large fixed costs that must be covered regardless of the size of the potential market. Consequently, large pharmaceutical companies are interested in developing new products primarily for sizable markets, for example, those with potential sales of approximately $50 million or more annually. Except for the pill and condoms, most contraceptive products have smaller markets than that. For example, in 1984 IUD sales in the United States were estimated to be less than $30 million dollars. Some pharmaceutical industry experts see little prospect for significant advances in new contraceptive methods likely to serve a large market in the United States and, therefore, to generate a substantial profit. Some executives at large drug companies do not believe that the relatively small markets they see for most of the proposed contraceptive innovations justify the substantial costs that would be required to develop the new products, and they want to avoid the liability risks and controversy associated with contraceptive products.

Public-sector funding and the increased activity of nonprofit groups and small entrepreneurial firms to some extent have substituted for the contraceptive-related research and development once performed by the large pharmaceutical firms. The growth of new research centers represents an important adjustment to declining pharmaceutical industry support for contraceptive research. Indeed, although increased involvement from large pharmaceutical companies would surely have an effect, that effect might not be immediately evident because of the relatively long time it takes before research leads to new products. However, because large pharmaceutical firms would have greater experience and more resources to evaluate, produce, and market products once they were available, the return of large companies might indeed increase the speed with which new products are introduced into widespread use.

Small Firms

With the decline in the number of large pharmaceutical companies involved in contraceptive development, there has been an increase in the number of small firms and R&D companies active in the field. Between 1970 and 1985, at least a dozen small companies became involved in the development of new contraceptives. One of the most successful of these companies was VLI Corp., which was established in 1976 and developed and marketed the Today contraceptive sponge. (The company has since been sold to Whitehall Laboratories, a division of American Home Products.) Most of these small companies rely on a combination of public and private sources to fund their research and development. A few depend entirely on government contracts and grants, while others fund their activities based on licensing agreements with large drug companies.

Stolle Research and Development Corporation is a particularly interesting example of the complex network that contraceptive development firms use to support their work. For its research on a 90-day injectable contraceptive, Stolle is collaborating with both Ortho Pharmaceutical Corp. and Family Health International. At the same time, the company is being funded through the AID-supported Contraceptive Research and Development Program at Eastern Virginia Medical School, to conduct research on a 30-day injectable contraceptive for women, a 90-day injectable contraceptive for men, and a 90-day injectable contraceptive microsphere for breastfeeding women. In conjunction with a project it supports at Ohio State University, WHO is funding Stolle to develop a one-year injectable vaccine for women. Some of these products will be licensed through Ortho Pharmaceutical Corp. or other large companies. Stolle does not plan to be directly involved in the marketing of products it develops.

GynoPharma, Inc., which was formed in 1984, is another small firm that is marketing and introducing new contraceptive products, such as the ParaGard copper IUD, which it introduced to the U.S. market in 1988. Unlike Stolle and GynoPharma, which work with a variety of partners to develop a range of products, many smaller contraceptive R&D companies are trying to develop a single technology that they hope to license to a large firm for marketing. For example, Endocon is working on biodegradable pellets. Small firms like VLI Corp., which developed the contraceptive sponge, may occasionally manufacture their products and, as happened with VLI, small firms with successful products may eventually be bought by large firms.

Whether working on a single product or on several products, most small firms are pursuing new methods for niche markets in the United States, although executives of these firms often believe their products, if successfully developed, could serve a mass market in the United States or abroad. In addition, as the data in the appendix show, with government or foundation funding, some small firms are also working on methods appropriate for less developed countries. Because small firms have fewer products and have usually invested a great deal of time, money, and research effort into the products they develop, they are more willing to risk the liability and possible adverse publicity associated with contraceptives than many of the larger, more diversified pharmaceutical companies, which stand to lose more financially if there is a public outcry against one of their products.

Companies such as Watson Laboratories and Lexis Pharmaceuticals Inc., which produce generic drugs, have also entered the contraceptive business, but their primary goal is to produce generic oral contraceptives rather than to develop new technology. However, one firm, Gynex Inc., which is marketing a generic oral contraceptive and other generic products, hopes to develop a contraceptive administered sublingually (corporate information memorandum, Gynex Inc., April 19, 1988).

Universities

Scientists at more than two dozen U.S. universities currently conduct applied research on potential new contraceptive methods with funds from NIH, AID (administered by the CONRAD program), and private foundations. In addition, special programs at a few universities have assumed responsibility for coordinating studies being carried out elsewhere; thus they serve as intermediary funders by providing support to researchers at other universities who become, in effect, grantees of the first university. This is the case with AID-funded programs at Eastern Virginia Medical School (CONRAD) and Georgetown University

(IISNFP), and previously it was the case at the Program for Applied Research in Fertility Regulation (PARFR) at Northwestern University. All these programs were funded by AID to conduct in-house research and to fund research done by others.

University scientists are a vital link in the chain of contraceptive development activities. All the organizations involved in the development of new fertility control technology depend in some way on the expertise of university-based scientists. They are a source of ideas and product concepts, and they frequently assist in evaluating new technology. There are, however, a range of potential conflicts among university scientists and corporate and nonprofit executives that limit the opportunities for successful long-term collaboration.

University scientists typically focus on basic research on biological processes and the publication of their results in scientific journals, not on applied research and product development. It is advances in basic research that bring them prestige and financial support. Such scientists may resist the limits imposed on their freedom to study whatever they wish, using whatever methods they prefer, when they participate in collaborative efforts in contraceptive development. Some collaborative arrangements with industry may also require a level of secrecy, which university-based scientists may find difficult to accept. Although the steadily increasing bureaucratization of university research has narrowed the differences between the norms of university and industry researchers, differences still exist that may limit effective collaboration.

Nonprofit Organizations

Although nonprofit organizations lack the capital as well as the technical and drug development expertise found in the largest for-profit companies, they are playing an increasingly important role in developing new contraceptive products and bringing them to market. To some extent, the cluster of donor agencies and nonprofit organizations working with university scientists and clinical researchers in the United States and abroad offers a functional equivalent of a large drug company, although some important gaps still exist in the ability of these groups to develop and market new products.

The Population Council and Family Health International (FHI) are the most important nonprofit organizations involved in contraceptive research and development in the United States. Together they spend more than $10 million annually studying new contraceptive products (Family Health International, 1988; Population Council, 1988; U.S. Agency for International Development, 1989). The mission of these organizations is to meet a social need rather than to make a profit. The research they support is oriented toward contraceptive products for developing countries and emphasizes products that try to better meet users' needs, including the needs of special groups, even if the particular product may be only marginally profitable.

The nonprofit research organizations rely primarily on the federal government, and to a lesser extent on foundations and occasionally on industry, for funding. They depend on drug and device manufacturers to mass produce the products they develop. Nonprofit organizations, such as the Population Council and FHI, perform a wide variety of tasks related to the development process. However, the specific tasks vary depending on the organization.

The program of the Population Council is the most comprehensive. It has its own research laboratories and animal facility on the campus of Rockefeller University in New York City, where it conducts basic research of a type not undertaken by other nonprofit groups. It also tests the new products it develops in the clinics of the International Committee for Contraception Research and registers those products for use throughout the world. FHI concentrates on the coordination of clinical evaluations of promising new contraceptive innovations initially developed by others. In some ways, FHI functions as a general contractor, coordinating the work of other specialists and groups. The Population Council and FHI work closely together on some projects. FHI is, for example, supporting some Phase III clinical trials of NORPLANT® contraceptive implants originally developed by the Population Council.

The activities of nonprofit organizations do not end with the development of a new method. The Population Council and Family Health International have both devoted some attention to introducing new methods. In addition, PATH, the Seattle-based nonprofit Program for Appropriate Technology in Health, was established in 1975 to facilitate the introduction of new and existing contraceptive technology in developing countries. PATH has assisted the Population Council and the World Health Organization in efforts to introduce new contraceptive technologies developed under their auspices. The Association for Voluntary Surgical Contraception as well as several Planned Parenthood affiliates are also among those who have helped to introduce new methods in specific circumstances.

Avenues to transfer the knowledge gained from contraceptive research to specialty companies or large pharmaceutical firms in order that they can market new contraceptive products need to be developed further. Links between contraceptive development and marketing are especially weak. There are examples of for-profit (VLI and the Today contraceptive sponge) and nonprofit (the Population Council and the NORPLANT® contraceptive implant) organizations successfully developing new contraceptives. But the development of these products, while driven by particular organizations, also required the collaboration of government, nonprofit groups, and for-profit institutions for successful manufacturing, distribution, and marketing.

As nonprofit organizations become more involved in contraceptive development, they face transition problems. An illustration is provided by the development of NORPLANT®. It was almost 20 years after the NORPLANT® concept was first proposed that the Population Council, which originated the technology, filed for FDA approval. A large pharmaceutical company that routinely processes a number of new drug applications would probably have been better equipped to complete the regulatory requirements associated with a new product in a more timely manner. Nonprofit organizations will continue to need considerable financial, personnel, and technical resources to successfully develop new products, in part because there is an organizational learning curve that means new organizational actors need time to master the tasks involved in the development process.

After the completion of early clinical tests, the Population Council looked for a company to manufacture the NORPLANT® system. Leiras Pharmaceuticals in Finland was approached and agreed to manufacture NORPLANT®. Wyeth Laboratories, the pharmaceutical company that holds the patent on levonorgestrel, the active ingredient in NORPLANT®, had assisted the Population Council in making its NDA submission to the FDA by providing access to clinical and toxicological data on levonorgestrel; although Wyeth had what amounted to the right of first refusal on manufacturing, it agreed to the Leiras arrangement. Wyeth holds the rights to market NORPLANT® in the United States and, pending the outcome of the complete FDA review and the results of the company's marketing surveys, it may exercise those rights. However, until the product was favorably recommended by an FDA advisory committee in April 1989, Wyeth's plans for marketing NORPLANT® were not widely known.

Also important is the problem some nonprofit organizations apparently have in recruiting high-quality scientific staff. These groups are at a particular disadvantage because they cannot offer their employees the financial rewards that industry can provide, nor can they offer the prestige, freedom, and security that university appointments provide. The problems nonprofit organizations have in attracting scientists are compounded by the short-term nature of most of their funding. These circumstances have led a mission-oriented federal agency like AID to rely on a funding arrangement such as CONRAD, which provides a mechanism for involving university-based scientists in the agency's contraceptive development program.

Several contraceptive products currently being developed commercially in the United States and Europe, such as copper IUDs and contraceptive implants, were originally investigated by nonprofit organizations. The drug companies that are now developing these products have become involved in part because the costs of much of the needed research have already been paid. The companies have an opportunity to earn a larger return than if they had had to pay for all the development costs. As long as the nonprofit sector is successfully completing much of the needed research, demonstrating the feasibility as well as the safety and probable appeal of new product concepts, and making this information publicly available, for-profit organizations are better off waiting for these results and then developing and marketing the most promising innovations.

Government and Private Funding Organizations

Through the funding of contraceptive research and development, the government and private foundations exercise considerable influence. (Chapter 6 discusses the funding provided by federal agencies and private organizations.) There are differences in what each group will support, based largely on the organization's goals and its particular history. The National Institutes of Health are oriented toward needs in the United States, while the Agency for International Development is eager to find a new technology that would serve the needs of the developing world better than existing products. Clearly, however, there is substantial overlap in these needs. NIH provides a much larger proportion of its support for basic research than AID, whose program is focused almost exclusively on applied research to develop new methods. Increasingly, however, AID and NIH provide support for the same people working on the same technologies.

The Ford, Rockefeller, and Andrew W. Mellon foundations have also been important sources of support for contraceptive development. Ford, however, withdrew from the field in 1983 and is unlikely to return. Both the Mellon and Rockefeller foundations have recently appointed new presidents, and at this writing are evaluating their programs and a range of new opportunities. At this stage, the level of future support for contraceptive development from these foundations is not clear.

From the viewpoint of those in the contraceptive development field, the support provided by the Ford, Rockefeller, and Mellon foundations has been particularly important because it has given researchers the flexibility to pursue new leads in a way that government support would not allow. For a time in the late 1970s, for example, researchers were not allowed to use AID money for collaborative contraceptive research projects in Chile, despite the international renown of Chilean contraceptive researchers; during that time, foundations provided funds that could be used to support collaborative work in Chile.

The World Health Organization

The World Health Organization is involved in the contraceptive development process mainly through the Special Programme in Research, Development, and Research Training in Human Reproduction (HRP). It is administered by WHO and cosponsored by WHO, the United Nations Development Programme (UNDP), the United Nations Fund for Population Activities (UNFPA), and the World Bank. HRP is actively involved in the development of new contraceptives and, through its method-related task forces, plays an important role in all phases of the development process, from preclinical research to introductory trials of newly developed products. HRP also helps strengthen research resources in less developed countries by providing financial and technical support for research institutions and for training in fields related to human reproduction. In addition, HRP issues guidelines for the clinical testing of new contraceptives, sponsors workshops on the safety of new drugs, and assists countries wishing to establish postmarketing surveillance systems for new contraceptives. HRP provides support to numerous clinical and research establishments, collaborates with clinical investigators in the United States and many other developed and developing countries in studying new contraceptive technologies, and works with government regulatory agencies, pharmaceutical firms, and nonprofit organizations involved in contraceptive development. Although the United States is a member of WHO, and U.S. scientists have for years worked closely with HRP, the United States has provided direct financial support to HRP for only two years since it was founded in 1972.

Two products, a new monthly injectable and a vaginal ring, have been developed under HRP auspices, and introductory trials of these products has begun in several developing countries. HRP is working closely with the nonprofit organization, PATH, which is helping WHO introduce these new contraceptives into developing country family planning programs, working with local pharmaceutical companies, drug regulatory officials, government policy makers, donor agencies, family planning program managers, clinicians, and potential users.

COLLABORATIVE EFFORTS IN CONTRACEPTIVE DEVELOPMENT

International and national organizations, including universities, nonprofit groups, and commercial firms, are increasingly collaborating on specific contraceptive development projects. Collaborative relationships link public and private organizations, funding agencies, basic research facilities, university-based scientists, clinical trials organizations, and large and small pharmaceutical companies.

The departure of a number of large pharmaceutical companies from contraceptive research and development activities in the United States increased the need for more collaborative efforts among the various organizations remaining in the field. Such collaborative efforts have also increased in recent years in part in an effort to reduce the costs and accelerate the pace of development. In many instances, collaboration is also a practical necessity because no one organization can successfully carry out the variety of tasks required to discover, develop, test, obtain approval for, and market a new contraceptive product.

There are several examples of collaboration in the development and introduction of new contraceptive methods. Development of the Today contraceptive sponge involved the developer, VLI Corp., two federal agencies, AID and NIH, which supported the nonprofit group FHI to evaluate the sponge by private physicians and clinics across the country and at several sites abroad. Development of injectable microspheres has involved AID and NIH, Ortho Pharmaceutical Corp., WHO, CONRAD, FHI, and Stolle Research and Development Corporation. The development, testing, and introduction of the NORPLANT® contraceptive implant has involved the Population Council, FHI, PATH, Wyeth-Ayerst Laboratories, and Leiras Pharmaceuticals, together with numerous individual clinical researchers around the world. The work was funded by AID, the International Development Research Centre of Canada, the Rockefeller Foundation, and several other sources. Ortho Pharmaceutical Corp. has supported basic research on inhibin at the University of Maryland at Baltimore. Ortho has also supported research on LHRH analogues at the Salk Institute and at Stolle Research and Development

Corporation. In 1989 the Population Council joined with the private Vastech Medical Products, Inc., to develop a new nonsurgical vasectomy device. In most of these collaborative efforts, each organization involved plays a distinct role, performing a separate function or carrying out a particular phase of development (see Atkinson et al., 1985). In other cases, however, because of funding constraints and existing institutional relationships, two organizations may conduct or support the same type of activity in different countries.

To be efficient and successful, collaborative efforts require careful planning, communication, and coordination. Financial, legal, scientific, medical, and regulatory issues and responsibilities need to be clearly defined. Management and funding problems, inadequate planning, and work delays within one organization can have a compounding effect, slowing the entire development process and adding to the costs of development. Delays in the introduction of NORPLANT®, for example, have resulted from such a combination of problems, including a lack of coordination between organizations and funding, regulatory, and product design problems.

Industry-University Collaboration

University scientists conducting basic research in biomedical laboratories funded mostly by the federal government often recognize the commercial potential of their studies of reproductive biology and fertility regulation, but they lack the resources needed to develop these ideas and to market innovations. Pharmaceutical companies, by contrast, have the needed resources and are almost always on the lookout for discoveries with commercial potential. This common set of interests often leads to university-industry collaboration.

The relationships that have evolved between pharmaceutical corporations and universities are as diverse as the individuals and institutions involved. Collaboration may involve the hiring of one consultant from a university by a particular company (or vice versa), or it may involve several universities and one or more companies working closely together on a project.

It is impossible to determine exactly how much money the pharmaceutical industry provides to universities for contraceptive research and development. With the abandonment of contraceptive R&D efforts by most pharmaceutical companies, industry's support of university-based research on new contraceptives has almost certainly declined in real terms. However, precise data on trends in this area are not available.

Despite problems, such as disputes over the granting of patent rights, the advantages of university-industry collaboration appear to outweigh the disadvantages. Universities' greater flexibility permits researchers to pursue interests that industry cannot support. Industry benefits from the discoveries generated from this research and from the expertise of highly trained university scientists.

Competitive Aspects of Contraceptive Development

The foundation of a pharmaceutical company's competitive advantage is that company's ability to discover and market new and useful products. The quest for innovative products is spurred by the potential demand for such products and, thus, the product's potential profitability. Some contraceptive products, such as oral contraceptives, have been very profitable, both in terms of a company's income and individual scientists' reputations. The competition characteristic of the drug industry leads to a great deal of secrecy about R&D efforts. The protection offered by trade secrets, the patent system, and market exclusivity rights makes secrecy essential in maintaining a competitive advantage. However, this need for secrecy also discourages collaboration and the open exchange of information on new discoveries. Time is another important factor in one company's ability to maintain a competitive edge over other companies. The company that gets a patent, FDA approval, or a product on the market first has a significant advantage in making a profit. Because many executives fear collaboration will slow development, they opt for doing as much of the research and development as possible within the company itself.

Competition also exists among small firms, nonprofit organizations, and scientists involved in contraceptive development. This competition involves efforts to secure the limited public and foundation funds available for contraceptive development and for the financial and professional rewards derived from new discoveries, published results, and patented products. The scientists and organization executives involved in contraceptive development must contend with conflicting goals. On one hand, they want and need successful collaborative relationships. On the other hand, they must frequently act in a way that threatens collaboration. They want to take credit for as many achievements as possible and reject association with as many problems as possible in order to ensure continued, ideally increasing, financial support and scientific recognition. This is not, of course, an uncommon problem in science, but it does make cordial long-term relationships difficult.

International Collaboration

Contraceptive development programs funded by national governments, such as those supported by NIH in the United States or by the national medical research councils in Europe, tend to focus on national needs and to support research conducted within the country. Research programs funded by WHO, by foreign assistance agencies such as AID, and by private foundations tend to be multicountry enterprises. International funding gives researchers the advantage of being able to work in countries with different legal and regulatory customs as well as with different research resources and different family planning environments. International collaboration may result in the development of a more diverse range of contraceptives at a faster pace than would be possible if research were conducted only within a specific country (Bardin, 1987).

STRENGTHENING THE PROCESS OF CONTRACEPTIVE DEVELOPMENT

Developing Country Institutions

Despite their more limited financial and technological resources, scientists in several developing countries, among them China, India, and Chile, have contributed to the development of new fertility regulating methods. Greep (1979), Kessler (1983), Free et al. (1983), and Segal (1987) have argued that developing countries could play a larger role in contraceptive development. Such a role would require that developing countries obtain additional financial and technical resources including laboratories, equipment, and doctorate-level scientists.

Scientists in less developed countries may be able to pursue contraceptive innovations that would more adequately meet the needs of people in those countries (Greep, 1979). Conducting contraceptive research in developing countries has the advantage that the testing of new products is done under the social and medical conditions and in the populations in which these new technologies would be used. Ethnic and geographic differences in users' reactions to new contraceptives, as well as the interaction of contraceptive products with diseases endemic to specific areas, demonstrate the utility of developing and testing new contraceptives in a variety of both developed and developing country settings (Adadevoh, 1983).

Over 60 clinical and research organizations in developing countries have already received institutional support from the World Health Organization's Special Programme of Research, Development, and Research Training in Human Reproduction (Adadevoh, 1983). Through collaborative research grants and contracts, Family Health International and the Population Council have also contributed to the support of scientists active in contraceptive research in developing countries. The Population Council has also provided fellowships for graduate training in fields related to contraceptive development. These efforts have helped many developing country institutions gain greater self-reliance, better research facilities, and an improved ability to conduct research (Adadevoh, 1983).

Although external technical and financial assistance is important, a national commitment to contraceptive R&D efforts is also essential to ensure a successful long-term development program. Government policies create the legal, regulatory, and economic environment that hinders or enhances contraceptive development efforts by private industry or by publicly supported groups. India, for example, has recently made changes in policy that should help to encourage collaborative efforts in contraceptive development and the local production of contraceptives (Program for Applied Technology and Health, 1988). Other countries could benefit from following India's example.

National Scientific Centers in the United States

In his 1987 State of the Union Address, President Reagan proposed the establishment of science and technology centers by federal research agencies; the National Science Foundation (NSF) began to support such centers in 1988. To help to integrate this new program with the NSF's existing current research programs, the President proposed substantial increases in the NSF budget.

Some people believe that the establishment of a national center for research on human reproduction and contraceptive development supported under the sciences and technology centers program could be an important change in the current organizational arrangements in the field of contraceptive development. In 1984 Congressman Jim Moody introduced a bill (H.R. 5335) to establish a National Institute on Population and Human Reproduction. However, given the successful collaboration already under way among contraceptive developers and clinical researchers, a more fruitful approach may be to strengthen the already functioning Contraceptive Development Branch of the Center for Population Research at the National Institute of Child Health and Human Development rather than establish either a new national center for research on human reproduction and contraceptive development or a new NIH institute.

CONCLUSION

The organization of contraceptive research and development in the United States has changed dramatically over the past two decades. In the early 1960s, most contraceptive research and development activities were sponsored and carried out by large pharmaceutical companies. By the 1980s, the government, small single-purpose companies, and nonprofit organizations had taken over most of the contraceptive-related research conducted in the United States. Increased government funding of contraceptive development in the early 1970s meant an expansion of the role of the public sector. Because most donors are particularly interested in research likely to have an impact in the developing world, research and development is increasingly being carried out by universities and nonprofit organizations that have strong international networks.

For the foreseeable future, much, perhaps most, of the cost of contraceptive research and method development will continue to be borne by government and private foundations. New contraceptive breakthroughs will require that universities and nonprofit organizations continue their development efforts. This may create temporary inefficiencies, delays, and added costs as these groups master the skills required to successfully develop and introduce new contraceptive products. Although most large pharmaceutical companies no longer see contraceptive development as sufficiently profitable, ways should be sought to increase collaboration between the pharmaceutical industry and the other organizations that remain active in the field.

APPENDIX TABLE 5.1 Organizations Currently Involved in Contraceptive Development

Type of Organization	Name of Organization	Projects/Products
U.S. GOVERNMENT AGENCIES	Agency for International Development (US AID), Office of Population	Funds support a spectrum of basic and applied research efforts, from basic biological research, to research on improvement of delivery systems, to training of service personnel
	National Institute of Child Health and Human Development (NICHD), Contraceptive Development Branch (CDB)	
U.S. NONPROFIT		
Nonspecialized research institutions	Research Triangle Institute (RTI)	Biodegradable polymers; delivery of contraceptive drugs
	SRI International	Biodegradable drug delivery systems for male and female fertility regulation
	Salk Institute	Peptide antagonists of LHRH as ovulation inhibitors
	Southern Research Institute	Long-acting LHRH microcapsule formulation; disposable diaphragm; male barrier device
Specialized contraceptive research institutions	Contraceptive Research and Development Program (CONRAD) at the Jones Institute, Eastern Virginia Medical School	Vaccine; NET microspheres; Shug vas deferens device; transdermal contraceptives
	Family Health International (FHI)	NET microspheres; biodegradable pellets; transdermals; plastic condoms; nonsurgical sterilization
	Institute for International Studies in Natural Family Planning (IISNFP) at Georgetown University	Natural family planning methods
	Population Council	Vaginal rings; LHRH analogues; inhibin; NORPLANT®; levonorgestrel-releasing IUD

72

APPENDIX TABLE 5.1 Continued

Type of Organization	Name of Organization	Projects/Products
Universities	Program for Appropriate Technology in Health (PATH)	Introduction and clinical training for monthly injectable; NORPLANT®
	Researchers at more than two dozen U.S. universities	Research and training in reproductive technology
U.S. FOR PROFIT		
Major Developer	Ortho Pharmaceutical Corporation	Injectables; microspheres; implants; LHRH antagonists; ovarian factors
Other Firms	ALZA Corporation	Progesterone IUD; oral-osmotic pill; transdermal controlled contraceptive
	Biotek, Inc.	Once-daily contraceptive skin patch
	Bivona Surgical Instruments	Shug vas deferens device
	Cygnus Research Corporation	Transdermal patch
	Endocon, Inc.	Biodegradable pellets
	Gynex, Inc.	Oral contraceptive
	GynoPharma, Inc.	Copper T-380 IUD; vaginal spermicide barrier; vaginal rings
	Hercon Laboratories Corporation	Transdermal patch
	Pacific Rim Bioscience Enterprises	Gossypol analogues
	Pharmetrix Corporation	Transdermal patches
	Stolle Research and Development Corporation	NET microspheres; male injectable 90-day microsphere; female contraceptive vaccine; contraceptive for breastfeeding women
	VLI Corporation (Whitehall Laboratories)	Today contraceptive sponge
	Vastech Medical Products, Inc.	Nonsurgical vasectomy device
	Wisconsin Pharmacal Company	Female condom

Category	Organization	Activities
U.S. PRIVATE FOUNDATIONS	Berlex Foundation	Limited support for research in reproductive biology
	Mellon Foundation	Support for contraceptive development, research, and training in reproductive sciences
	Rockefeller Foundation	Support for contraceptive development and research in reproductive sciences
INTERNATIONAL AGENCIES	International Development Research Centre (IDRC)	Support for contraceptive development activities
	International Organization for Chemical Synthesis in Development (IOCD)	Limited research on new chemical entities for fertility regulation
	United Nations Fund for Population Activities (UNFPA)	Support for contraceptive development activities
	World Bank	Support for WHO contraceptive development program
	WHO Special Programme in Research, Development, and Research Training in Human Reproduction (HRP)	Vaginal rings; injectables; vaccines; postovulatory methods; ovulation detection and prediction
NATIONAL RESEARCH CENTERS IN DEVELOPING COUNTRIES	Indian Council of Medical Research	Injectables; vaccines
	National Research Institute for Family Planning (People's Republic of China)	Once-a-month pills; long-acting injectables; vaginal rings; gossypol; prostaglandins; spermicidal agents
NON-U.S. PHARMACEUTICAL FIRMS	FEMCARE Ltd. (England)	Filshie clip

APPENDIX TABLE 5.1 Continued

Type of Organization	Name of Organization	Projects/Products
	Lamberts Ltd. (England)	Prentif cavity-rim cervical cap, Dumas cap; Vimule cap
	Leiras Pharmaceuticals (Finland)	NORPLANT® contraceptive implant
	Organon International (The Netherlands)	Implants; vaginal rings; contraceptive steroids
	Roussel Uclaf (France)	RU-486
	(subsidiary of Hoechst Pharmaceuticals)	
	Schering, AG (West Germany)	Contraceptive steroids

Note: This table is intended to illustrate the range of organizations active in the contraceptive development field as well as the range of products being studied. Information was obtained from annual reports, published materials on contraceptives, and telephone conversations with staff at pharmaceutical firms and research institutions. Some organizations and/or contraceptive development projects may have been omitted inadvertently or have been omitted because the information was unavailable because of the proprietary nature of contraceptive development. This table is illustrative and is not meant to be an endorsement of any group or product by the National Academy of Sciences.

6

Funding for
Contraceptive Development

Fostering creativity and stimulating innovation in the field of contraceptive development depends on the training and employment of creative people; on steady financial support and, therefore a stable working environment; on the timely funding of promising new ideas; on support for cross-disciplinary and international collaboration; and on the ability to provide scientists with personal recognition and rewards (Westwood and Sekine, 1988). This chapter examines the resources that are currently available to make these things happen. We present data on trends in the funding of contraceptive development and of basic research in reproductive biology and review the support provided by the National Institutes of Health (NIH), the Agency for International Development (AID), private foundations, as well as pharmaceutical companies and venture capitalists. Unfortunately, data are not available to measure the impact that federal and private funding of contraceptive development has had on the frequency of innovation or to determine the exact level of funding necessary to bring a promising new contraceptive to the market.

The first organized support of reproductive research in the United States was provided by the Rockefeller family in 1921, through the Committee on Research in Problems of Sex, which was organized by the National Academy of Sciences (Greep et al., 1976). The committee operated until 1963, when the National Institute of Child Health and Human Development (NICHD) was established and began funding research on human reproduction and contraceptive methods. With the creation of the Center for Population Research (CPR) at NICHD in 1968, and concomitant increased commitment to contraceptive research by the Office of Population at the Agency for International Development, federal support for

75

reproductive biology and contraceptive development increased substantially. Private foundations provided additional support for contraceptive development during the 1960s and 1970s. The drug industry also supported contraceptive R&D, which had been initiated in the 1950s with research on contraceptive steroids.

Around 1970, at least a half dozen large U.S. drug companies were each spending several million dollars annually on contraceptive research and development. Since that time, these companies have continued to market oral contraceptives and to study alternative formulations for them. But only Ortho Pharmaceutical Corp. has continued a significant research program aimed at developing new contraceptives for the American market.

Federal funding, which had increased significantly from the mid-1960s to the mid-1970s, did not continue to grow as fast as it had. The Ford Foundation, once a major supporter of research on reproductive biology and contraceptive development, withdrew from the field. While some new funds came from small firms or venture capitalists and from increases in AID's expenditure for contraceptive development, the trend was no longer steadily upward.

Today the funding of contraceptive development is a dynamic process in which funds flow in multiple directions, both to and from organizations involved in different phases of the contraceptive development process. The development of a new contraceptive is rarely funded by a single source. The federal government and private foundations fund basic research at universities. Results of this work may then be used by pharmaceutical firms, which conduct applied contraceptive R&D in their laboratories, by scientists working at nonprofit research organizations supported by AID, or by clinical investigators collaborating with the World Health Organization.

FUNDING FOR CONTRACEPTIVE DEVELOPMENT

Figure 6.1 provides a schematic representation of the flow of funds for contraceptive development. Funds generally move from government funding agencies and private foundations to university research centers, nonprofit research organizations, and small research firms. Some of the funds received by nonprofit organizations, such as Family Health International, the Population Council, and universities (as in the CONRAD program), are provided to researchers around the world and small R&D firms for work on the development of new contraceptives. Nonprofit organizations occasionally receive funds from other sources: for example, FHI receives funds from its for-profit subsidiary, Clinical Research International (CRI), and the Population Council uses funds from its endowment to support some contraceptive research. Although the magnitude is not known, some R&D funds also flow from large drug companies to small R&D firms, universities, and nonprofit research organizations involved in various stages of contraceptive development.

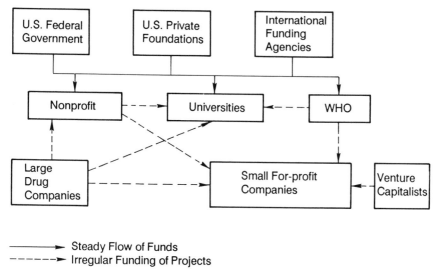

Steady Flow of Funds
Irregular Funding of Projects

FIGURE 6.1 Flow of funds for contraceptive development.

Many of the resources provided by American organizations are used outside the United States. The Rockefeller Foundation supports contraceptive development overseas, and FHI and the Population Council fund networks of clinical investigators and research centers around the world. U.S. contributions to the World Bank, the United Nations, and other organizations indirectly contribute to contraceptive development efforts in less developed countries. NIH's funding of contraceptive development, however, is confined largely to U.S. institutions.

Pharmaceutical Industry Funding

Our analysis of the funding of contraceptive research and development is incomplete because we have only a very limited picture of the pharmaceutical industry's contributions. Given the resources available and the proprietary nature of the information, the committee found it impossible to obtain reliable estimates of the amount of money being spent on research on reproductive biology or contraceptive development by American pharmaceutical firms. Data from the Pharmaceutical Manufacturers Association show that the U.S. drug industry's total R&D expenditures for all types of drugs combined—not simply those related to contraception—have increased steadily between 1970 and 1986, in both absolute dollars and as a percentage of total sales. This does not imply, however, that research expenditures for contraceptive R&D have increased.

The largest American pharmaceutical firm carrying out research on new contraceptives is Ortho Pharmaceutical Corporation, whose annual R&D budget was approximately $160 million in 1986. It is not known, however, how much of this went to contraceptive R&D. Ortho Pharmaceutical Corporation and a few European drug companies are currently supporting contraceptive research and development being conducted by smaller research firms, such as Stolle Research and Development Corporation, Endocon Corporation, and Cygnus Inc. ALZA Corporation is funding the development of new drug delivery systems (e.g., transdermal patches and oral osmotic pills), which may have applications in the field of hormonal contraception, but the amount of funds it allocates to these activities is not known. The extent to which other large drug companies fund research by small firms or at universities is also not known. Based on informal reports from scientists in the field and pharmaceutical industry executives, our judgment is that there has been a substantial decline in the amount of funding provided for contraceptive R&D on the part of the drug industry since the mid-1970s.

Quite often the small private firms involved in contraceptive development activities rely on initial funding from venture capital groups or individual private investors. However, in most cases, the details of these arrangements are not publicly known. Development of the Today contraceptive sponge, for example, was supported by venture capital. Contracap and Gynex, two companies presently developing contraceptive products, were initially funded by the same private investor before going public in 1983 and 1986, respectively.

Given the lack of data available on private organizations, this chapter concentrates on the public sector and foundation funding of contraceptive development. It should be clear, however, that large pharmaceutical firms are an important potential source of support for research and development related to new contraceptives.

Federal Funding

To analyze trends in government and foundation funding of contraceptive development and of basic research in reproductive biology in the United States, the committee relied primarily on the data collected and published annually by the National Institute of Child Health and Human Development through the Interagency Council on Population Research (ICPR).

In 1985 the Alan Guttmacher Institute (AGI) published a study examining the worldwide funding of contraceptive research and development between 1980 and 1983 (Atkinson et al., 1985). The AGI survey produced estimates of U.S. government funding that were lower than the figures provided by NIH for the same years. AGI estimates of government funding of basic research in reproductive biology are about half of those reported in NICHD and about 5 percent less than NIH estimates of government funding of contraceptive development. AGI estimates of foundation funding of basic research in reproductive biology and of contraceptive development are one-third less than the estimates reported by NICHD.

The main source of the differences between the NICHD and the AGI estimates are differences in the classification of projects as basic reproductive research or applied contraceptive development. For this report, we accept the broader definition of basic research in reproductive biology used by NICHD. NICHD divides basic research in reproductive biology into the following areas: development and function of the reproductive system; female fertility; male and female fertility; fertilization, including immediate prefertilization processes; preimplantation development; implantation; and reproductive endocrinology.

As defined by NICHD, contraceptive development includes research on drug syntheses and testing, drug delivery systems and oral formulations testing, vaginal and uterine contraceptive devices and drugs, and sterilization. Contraceptive development also includes studies of ". . . natural or synthetic agents other than presently used contraceptives, new contraceptive devices and reversible sterilization techniques" (National Institute of Child Health and Human Development, 1987:7).

There is no inherent bias in the sources of data NICHD used, and its methodology and criteria for classifying and categorizing projects appear to be sound. Furthermore, NICHD has collected data annually for nearly 20 years, making it possible to estimate long-term trends in funding. Researchers from AGI categorized projects on the basis of their titles, a procedure that is not a clear improvement. The NICHD may overestimate the amount of contraceptive-related research under way, especially since much of the reported basic biological research is not conducted with a contraceptive application in view (although such applications may result).

Table 6.1 presents data on the trend in the funding of research on reproductive biology and contraceptive development in constant 1973 dollars by the federal government and private foundations. Support for both basic research on reproductive biology and contraceptive development increased between 1973 and 1987. In current dollars, spending for reproductive biology research more than quadrupled, from $30 million in 1973 to $135 million in 1987; spending for contraceptive development grew from $7 million in 1973 to $36 million in 1987. In constant dollars, funding for reproductive biology research increased by 64 percent, from $30.2 million in 1973 to 49.5 million in 1987; funding for contraceptive development increased by 78 percent, from $7.4 million to $13.2 million.

Although the increases in funding have been substantial, the pattern of support concerns some of those in the contraceptive development field. An important source of the difference between the AGI and NICHD estimates of funding is based on the conclusion of the AGI researchers that "most fundamental nondirected research . . . does not contribute directly to the development of new methods" and so including funding for it "has tended to misleadingly suggest that the funds available for contraceptive development were larger than they actually were" (Atkinson et al., 1985:198). Atkinson and her colleagues note that there may be differences of opinion as to which category a particular research project should be assigned.

TABLE 6.1 Federal and Foundation Funding for Basic Research in Reproductive Biology and Contraceptive Development (fiscal years 1973-1987, in constant 1973 dollars—millions)

	Reproductive Biology				Contraceptive Development			
Year	Total[a]	HHS	AID	Foundations[b]	Total	AID	HHS	Foundations[b]
1973	30.2	22.8		6.7	7.4	2.9	3.2	1.3
1974	33.7	27.6		5.6	9.6	2.1	3.9	3.6
1975	29.7	24.5		4.7	10.3	2.8	5.1	2.3
1976	32.6	27.9		3.4	10.9	3.6	5.3	2.1
1977	29.9	25.6		3.3	14.1	5.3	5.4	3.3
1978	35.6	30.4		3.6	11.8	4.5	4.9	2.4
1979	38.5	33.1		3.6	11.2	4.8	4.5	1.8
1980	39.4	35.4		1.9	10.8	4.3	4.9	1.5
1981	43.1	39.0		2.0	10.6	3.5	4.8	2.3
1982	42.6	38.0		1.9	9.8	3.6	4.4	1.7
1983	44.5	40.8		1.3	9.5	3.4	4.4	1.7
1984	43.0	40.2		.8	9.0	4.5	3.1	1.4
1985	43.4	39.4		1.1	11.6	6.8	3.8	1.0
1986	43.6	38.4		1.5	12.3	7.3	3.6	1.4
1987	49.5	44.4		1.7	13.2	8.1	3.8	1.3

[a]Total includes other federal sources not shown separately in table.
[b]Population Council plus Ford, Rockefeller, and Mellon foundations.

Source: Unpublished data from the National Institute of Child Health and Human Development (NICHD), National Institutes of Health, Bethesda, Maryland.

The committee did not have the resources to conduct an independent review of the allocation of projects and so is not in a position to endorse either AGI's or the NICHD's Interagency Council on Population Research's allocation. That said, however, it is worth noting that many active in the contraceptive development field believe that the substantial increases shown in Table 6.1 are not an accurate reflection of the trend in funding for activities directly related to contraceptive development. Another factor in the funding trend for basic research in reproductive biology is the decline in foundation support for such work. The increase in support from NICHD and the decline in foundation support means that foundation funding now plays a very small role in supporting basic research in reproductive biology. In 1973, foundations accounted for about a fifth of all funding for basic research in reproductive biology; by 1987, foundations contributed less than 2 percent of all funds spent on basic biological research.

Funding for contraceptive development has also increased between 1973 and

1986, but it was always considerably less than the amount devoted to basic research. In most years for which data are available, the total spent on contraceptive development was between 25 and 30 percent of the total spent on basic research. Annual foundation funding for contraceptive development has been relatively stable throughout the 1980s, but at a lower level than in the 1970s. Funding from NICHD was relatively stable after declining from the highest years of 1975, 1976, and 1977. However, there was a sharp decline in NICHD funding of contraceptive development in 1984. Some of that loss has been made up in more recent years, but NICHD now provides more than $1.5 million less (in constant dollars) than it did in the mid-1970s.

The contributions of the Agency for International Development to the funding of contraceptive development have followed the pattern of NICHD; increases in funding occurred in the mid-1970s and declines took place in the early 1980s. Between 1983 and 1987, however, AID funding of contraceptive development increased by 138 percent (in constant dollars). It seems unlikely that such increases will continue, but the recent growth in federal funding for contraceptive development has given greater visibility to AID-funded organizations, such as Family Health International.

Basic research on reproductive biology has enjoyed the largest proportion of federal funding in the population sciences, and its share has been increasing. Since 1981 over 50 percent of all federal funding for population research has been channeled to basic research in reproductive biology. From 1974 to 1987 the proportion of federal dollars spent on basic research in reproductive biology has increased from 50 to 71 percent. Studies of reproductive endocrinology have dominated this research area and have consistently received 36 percent to 45 percent of all research funds allocated to reproductive biology.

Between 1973 and 1987 the National Institutes of Health provided over 90 percent of the money for research in reproductive biology. Funding of reproductive research by other federal agencies has not increased significantly in constant 1973 dollars over the past 14 years. The Environmental Protection Agency, which provided funding for research on reproductive biology from 1980 to 1985, discontinued funding in 1986. The Veterans Administration began funding research in reproductive biology in 1975 but discontinued reporting funding activity in 1981, although it still funds a small number of projects. The Department of Agriculture began funding population research in 1986; the major portion of its funds go to research in reproductive biology. The Department of Energy first funded research in reproductive biology in 1979, and the National Science Foundation has concentrated its population research funding in this area since 1981. Only AID and NICHD support contraceptive development.

The largest concentration of funds in contraceptive development has been for "general or multiple studies of contraceptives," because AID funds for clinical trials are included in this category. However, the largest number of projects has consistently been in the drug synthesis and testing category.

Foundation Funding

Since 1973 the Ford and Rockefeller foundations have provided information on their grants for research related to population and contraceptive development to the Interagency Committee on Population Research at NICHD. The Andrew W. Mellon Foundation began reporting in 1979.

The Ford Foundation began funding reproductive research and contraceptive development in the 1950s. The Rockefeller Foundation declared population to be one of its main areas of interest in 1963. The Mellon Foundation began funding population research in 1979, although it had previously supported the Population Council and the Planned Parenthood Federation. In 1980 the Ford, Rockefeller, and Mellon foundations established a collaborative contraceptive development research program in an effort to accelerate the development of new and improved contraceptives. In 1985, however, the Ford Foundation discontinued its program of support for contraceptive development.

Some of the Ford and Rockefeller funding is also reported to the ICPR by the Population Council. This happens because the Population Council is supported by grants from foundations (including Ford, Rockefeller, and Mellon), international organizations, and federal agencies (including AID and NICHD), which it then uses to support contraceptive development, most of which falls under the auspices of its International Committee for Contraception Research (ICCR). For this analysis, funds reported by the Population Council for contraceptive development and reproductive processes that come from other sources are attributed to the original donor, whether it was a private foundation or a federal agency. FHI, the CONRAD program, and other organizations that receive their funds from private foundations or federal agencies are treated in the same way as the Population Council.

Beginning in 1988, the John D. and Catherine T. MacArthur Foundation, the William and Flora Hewlett Foundation, and the Berlex Foundation were included in Interagency Committee on Population Research's annual survey. In 1987 the Berlex Foundation began providing fellowships for innovative research in reproductive medicine, including contraceptive and fertility-related research. Although the MacArthur, Hewlett, and David and Lucile Packard foundations support family planning programs, they have not supported contraceptive development.

In the early 1970s, private foundation funding provided for population research was concentrated on support to studies of reproductive biology; only 10 percent went to support contraceptive development activities. During the 1980s, foundation funding for reproductive biology has decreased and now represents about 10 percent of all the foundation funding for population. The proportion allocated to contraceptive development tripled, going from 10 percent in 1973 to 29 percent in 1977; however, it has since declined and in 1985, the last year for which data are available, was at approximately the level it had been in the early 1970s. At the same time these changes were taking place, the proportion of foundation support allocated to research in the social and behavioral sciences related to population more than doubled, from 25 percent in 1973 to 60 percent in 1985.

Funding Worldwide

The annual inventories of funding for population-related research published by the Interagency Council on Population Research provide data only on funding provided by U.S. government agencies and private foundations. It has been estimated that the United States is the source of approximately 75 percent of the worldwide funding for reproductive research and contraceptive development (Atkinson et al., 1985). To provide an indication of the trends in funding outside the United States, we have relied on studies by Greep (1979), Greep et al. (1976), and Atkinson et al. (1980, 1985), which provide the most complete account of the levels and sources of worldwide funding for contraceptive development. Unfortunately, the most recent of these studies reports on trends only to 1983. Moreover, as noted above, the data provided by Atkinson et al. are a lower estimate of the financial support provided by the U.S. government than are the data presented earlier in this report.

After reaching a peak in 1972, annual worldwide funding for contraceptive development dropped sharply in 1975 (Lincoln and Kaeser, 1987). Between 1977 and 1983, funding remained at a relatively constant level. Moreover, support for contraceptive development from developed countries other than the United States has been declining in both current and constant dollars since the late 1970s (Atkinson et al., 1985).

During 1980-1983, the average annual worldwide expenditure on basic reproductive research and contraceptive development was approximately $154 million, of which an estimated $63 million was spent for contraceptive development. This figure includes funding for the evaluation of long-term safety of existing methods (Atkinson et al., 1985). Less developed countries contributed only about 1 percent of these funds. A few developing countries, such as China, India, Chile, Mexico, and Brazil (Atkinson, 1985), have made significant contributions, but most other developing countries have not.

Atkinson et al. estimate that private industry spent an estimated $22 million or about 35 percent of the total provided for contraceptive development, and seven specialized contraceptive development organizations spent an estimated $26 million or 41 percent of worldwide expenditures for contraceptive development. The remaining 24 percent of expenditures was provided mainly by national governments that funded mission-oriented research projects.

World Health Organization

Between 1970 and 1980, support for the World Health Organization's Special Programme on Human Reproduction increased steadily from about $1 million to almost $20 million. From 1980 to 1984, funds dropped to $13 million. Since then, funding has increased to more than $20 million in 1987, of which about $9 million was allocated for the development of new contraceptives (WHO, 1987). In 1987 the World Bank began to provide direct financial support to HRP, with an initial contribution of $2 million. The United Nations Development Programme, the World Bank, and the United Nations Fund for Population Activities joined WHO in sponsoring HRP in 1987. Of the more than $182 million provided between 1970 and 1986 to the Human Reproduction Programme (WHO, 1987) by national governments and other donors, the United States contributed only $3.2 million in two installments, the first in 1980–1981 for $3 million, and the second in 1986 for $165,000.

The level of American support for HRP reflects a statutory prohibition against donations to HRP passed by Congress in 1982 and justified on the grounds that it was necessary to shift funding from contraceptive development toward service delivery. In 1986 the prohibition was repealed and $165,000 was given to HRP. Since then, no additional funds have been provided by the United States. However, some of the support HRP receives from WHO, the United Nations Development Programme, and the World Bank takes advantage of the U.S. contributions to these organizations. Sweden (which gave $73 million), Norway (which gave $26 million), United Kingdom ($24 million), the United Nations Fund for Population Activities ($17 million), Denmark ($13 million), and Canada ($8 million) were the largest contributors to HRP during the 1970–1986 period.

TRAINING

The training of scientists in reproductive biology and fields related to contraceptive development is considered by many experts to be of prime importance for continued advances in the field. It usually takes three to six years to complete the training necessary for a career in basic reproductive research or applied contraceptive development. Declining or sporadic funding from foundations and government agencies contributes to a reduction of the number of scientists who are being trained in the field of reproductive biology and contraceptive development. The lessened interest of most pharmaceutical companies also contributes to a lack of opportunities in the field. The decision to go into a particular field depends on expected career opportunities after training, and the costs of going through training. While the costs of training have risen in recent years, the expected benefits and career opportunities have fallen.

The Ford and Rockefeller foundations supported training programs in the 1950s and 1960s. Although the Rockefeller Foundation continues to support some training, in recent years the National Institutes of Health and the Andrew W. Mellon Foundation have been the major source of funds for training in reproductive biology and contraceptive development in the United States. However, NIH funding for training in the reproductive sciences has fluctuated. Between 1970 and 1987, predoctoral NIH fellowship grants ranged from 48 to 100 per year, while postdoctoral NIH fellowships in the reproductive sciences ranged from 37 to 68 per year. Between 1970 and 1987, NIH faculty fellow awards in reproductive sciences ranged from a low of 8 awards in 1973 to a high of 61 awards in 1979, to 37 awards in 1987.

Between 1975 and 1985, 208 people were trained in the reproductive sciences with support from Mellon's fellowship program. There was an increase in the number of Mellon fellowships awarded, from 2 in 1975 to a peak number of 101 in 1982. However, the number of fellowships declined to 86 in 1985. Most of the Mellon fellowships have been to postdoctoral researchers (71 percent) and faculty fellows (28 percent).

Although the reduced pool of scientific personnel in this area and the decline of fellowship awards may be the result of a decrease in demand, the converse may also be true: a reduction in available personnel may be contributing to the decline in contraceptive research and development. Expanding the research output of any science requires an adequate number of trained people working in the field. Training programs are essential to ensure long-term increases in scientific output; it is therefore important to support training for the nation's scientists. Reproductive biology and contraceptive development must compete with other research areas for funds for training. Allocation of additional funds for training in these areas would demonstrate greater national commitment to this field.

The training of scientists in human reproduction and contraceptive development and the supply of scientists who continue to work in this field is also influenced by the availability of good jobs and the prospects of support for research in contraceptive research. The sensitive and sometimes publicly controversial nature of contraceptive research has probably made the field less attractive. The recent focus of public attention and scientific research interest on AIDS, on new biotechnology, and on genetic engineering, as well as the increased funding and research opportunities in these areas, together with the pharmaceutical industry's interest in programs to develop new drugs for degenerative diseases may also be diverting some scientists from the field of contraceptive development.

The decline in the number of training grants in the reproductive sciences during the 1980s, combined with the other factors that have reduced the number of people entering the field, has led to a concern about the aging of scientists active in contraceptive development. One important consequence of the limited number of researchers involved in contraceptive development is an undesirable thinness in this field, resulting in a sparse literature on each new contraceptive method (Segal, 1989). Replications of clinical studies are needed but often not done because of the limited financial and human resources available.

The limits of the field's resources and the steadily increasing cost of scientific equipment have created another problem that is often overlooked in discussions of the prospects for new methods. New areas of contraceptive research will require even more sophisticated equipment and research laboratories than ever before. As contraceptive development moves in the direction of new biotechnology, genetic engineering, and molecular biology, more complex equipment will be required. The need for state-of-the-art technology in university laboratories and in the contraceptive development field will cause R&D costs to grow, as research organizations attempt to keep up with higher and higher scientific standards.

In 1976, Greep and his collaborators estimated that between 2,500 and 3,000 scientists were actively involved in research on reproduction and contraceptive development in 419 institutions worldwide (Greep, 1979). The vast majority of the institutions where research and training were taking place were in developed countries. In the early 1960s the Ford Foundation, in an effort to expand the scientific infrastructure devoted to contraceptive development in developing countries, began supporting training in the field of reproductive and contraceptive research outside the United States. In more recent years, the World Health Organization's Human Reproduction Programme, recognizing the need to build training and institutional research capabilities in developing countries, has taken a leading role in these areas.

Medical research councils and foundations in some European countries and some developing countries also provide funds for training in basic reproductive research and contraceptive development. Unfortunately, we were unable to establish the amount spent on such activities. In the 1985 Alan Guttmacher Institute survey (Atkinson et al., 1985), for example, it is not possible to separate funding for training from support for basic research provided by developed countries other than the United States or by developing countries. But total expenditures for both training and research on reproductive biology outside the United States amounted to only 6 percent of the worldwide total expended in 1983—thus the contribution of these other countries is not large (Atkinson et al., 1985).

Although not a focus of this report, it is worth noting that the training needs of scientists in less developed countries appear particularly urgent. Declines in funding and dramatic increases in tuition in developed countries, where most such training is available, have not been compensated for by the increased availability of training opportunities in developing countries themselves. The net result of these changes appears to be a decrease in the number of scientists from less developed countries going abroad for Ph.D. training in research related to reproductive biology or contraceptive development (Kessler, 1983:185).

RECOMMENDATIONS

We believe that research in reproductive biology and contraceptive development is underfunded. Development of new contraceptive methods is expensive, and additional resources could accelerate the process of innovation. Federal funding in these areas should keep pace with the rising costs of research and development. With the decline in industry's support, NIH should consider increasing its funding of contraceptive development to help bridge the gap between basic research and the marketing of new contraceptives.

Although the contributions of the Rockefeller and Mellon foundations to contraceptive development in recent years have been significant, the committee encourages these and other private foundations to initiate, resume, or expand their support of applied contraceptive research and development. Nonprofit organizations involved in the costly process of bringing new contraceptive products through clinical testing, gaining regulatory approval, and helping introduce them to the market are in particular need of increased support. Long-term funding is particularly important for those involved in contraceptive development; to the extent possible, federal agencies and private foundations should provide long-term funding commitments.

If the nation wishes to increase the priority of research on reproductive biology and contraceptive development, it is important to increase the pool of young scientists entering the field. Several researchers told the committee that bright young scientists are attracted to other fields of research, in which more funding is available for fellowships and research. A special grants program for young scientists might attract new talent and encourage more innovative research in the fields of reproductive biology and contraceptive development. The committee recommends that NIH expand its training program in the reproductive sciences and contraceptive development, preferably at a high and predictable level. The Mellon Foundation training program has been successful and the committee recommends that other private foundations consider support for training. As part of an expanded effort to attract qualified people to this area of research, as well as to be more responsive to the contraceptive needs and concerns of women and minority groups, more women and more members of minority groups should be encouraged to enter the field of contraceptive development.

Continued support for contraceptive development and research training in other countries, particularly in the developing world, should be encouraged as part of a worldwide effort to help meet country-specific contraceptive needs. The United States should provide direct financial support to the WHO's Human Reproduction Programme to help achieve this goal.

CONCLUSION

In a recent review of funding for contraceptive development, Harkavy (1987) noted that levels of funding for contraceptive development have remained remarkably modest and uncertain and that "public sector R&D organizations have difficulty in obtaining substantial support from governmental and private donors because of impatience for short-term results, concern that small-scale operations are not effective, tensions between U.S. and European donors, and even ambivalence on the usefulness of new technology" (p. 307).

Federal funds for contraceptive development have remained virtually unchanged (in constant dollars) over the last decade, while pharmaceutical industry and private foundation support for contraceptive development has diminished. Although federal funds for research on reproductive processes has increased in constant dollars since the mid-1970s, private foundation support has declined substantially, and the loss of the industry's resources has been critical. Because of the decline in industry's support of contraceptive R&D and the limited amount and unpredictable character of foundation support, the federal government, through NIH and AID, has assumed an increasingly important funding role.

The committee believes that federal funding should keep pace with the rising costs of research and development. We believe that current funding arrangements in the contraceptive development field need to be reevaluated by those directly involved to determine whether they are the most useful, productive, and cost-effective allocation of funds and are most likely to lead to the development of new contraceptive methods.

We have not attempted to determine what allocation of funds would maximize productivity in the field of contraceptive development. Atkinson et al. (1985) estimated that a 75-percent increase in the annual total expenditures in contraceptive development from the 1985 level of $30 million by eight major contraceptive R&D organizations could significantly accelerate progress on new methods now under development. These estimates were based on the amounts said to be needed by executives for these groups in 1986–1988 to accelerate progress or to follow up new contraceptive leads (Atkinson et al., 1986). Although our judgment is that this estimate is low, we have not conducted a detailed assessment of the funds needed to develop and market the potential new methods discussed in Chapter 3.

Training grants in the reproductive sciences fluctuate widely from year to year, and there is a concern that the number of scientists actively involved in contraceptive development is very small and that the scientific literature on various new methods makes confirmation of the effectiveness and the risks and benefits of new methods difficult.

7

Regulation and
Contraceptive Development

This chapter briefly reviews the process of contraceptive development and examines the U.S. Food and Drug Administration (FDA) requirements and procedures for approving new contraceptive drugs and devices. It then compares them with those of regulatory bodies in other countries and those of the World Health Organization.

Some analysts contend that the regulatory climate in the United States has impeded the U.S. pharmaceutical industry's willingness to pursue innovations in contraceptive development (Isaacs and Holt, 1987a; Greep et al., 1976; Djerassi, 1987, 1981). Reports of the regulatory problems associated with contraceptive development tend to be anecdotal and not based on a systematic analysis of the regulatory environment. Nevertheless, a good deal is known about the impact of FDA and the patent and tax laws implemented and overseen by other U.S. government bodies on innovation in the pharmaceutical field. Some of what we know clearly applies to contraceptive development.

The FDA is a reviewer, not an initiator, of new products. Pharmaceutical or device firms, research groups, or government agencies conduct research and test new contraceptives and present their results to FDA for review. Drugs and medical devices are regulated separately and are reviewed by different units of the FDA, although the requirements are similar. A contraceptive vaccine would be regulated differently from a contraceptive drug or medical device; like other vaccines, it would be regulated as a biological product under §351 of the Public Health Service Act (42 U.S.C. §262 [1982 & Supp. 1988]; 21 C.F.R. pt. 600 [1988]).

FDA's requirements help protect people from potentially harmful products.

Yet the time, costs, and data required to gain approval of a new product reduce the incentives to undertake innovative research and may also reduce effective patent life and, thus, the profitability of new products. The balance between allowing ample opportunity to develop useful new products and protecting the safety of consumers is at the heart of the debate about the FDA's safety and effectiveness requirements for new drugs generally and for contraceptives in particular. For some, the FDA is regarded as a significant barrier to better contraceptive methods and therefore to fewer unwanted pregnancies and abortions. For others, the FDA's standards and procedures are seen as being not rigorous enough and too easily influenced by pressures from private industry.

THE DEVELOPMENT PROCESS

Contraceptive development involves identifying possible avenues to intervening in the reproductive process, eliminating those that are ineffective, infeasible, or unlikely to be acceptable because of side effects or for other reasons, then testing the remaining drugs or devices for safety and efficacy. Throughout this process, changes may be made in a method's composition, dosage, or mode of administration. Some changes may necessitate additional testing, and some tests may need to be replicated in different populations.

The development of a new contraceptive, like the development of other drugs and therapeutic devices, is a complex, multifaceted process involving a wide variety of scientific disciplines. Successful contraceptive development requires millions of dollars, takes years to complete, and may involve the testing of thousands of different chemical compounds. Many drug formulations are discarded during the development process because of concern about safety, efficacy, feasibility of delivery, or marketability. In drug development generally, FDA approval is sought for only 1 out of every 10,000 new chemicals synthesized in the laboratory. One study found that, of 20 new chemical entities identified as potential antifertility agents between 1963 and 1976, 17 were placed into human trials, but only 3 were submitted to FDA for approval, of which 2 were actually approved (Harper, 1983).

It is difficult to estimate the cost of developing a new contraceptive or any other new product because of the problems involved in incorporating the costs of false starts and opportunity costs in the calculations. One recent study (Wiggins, 1987) estimates that it cost $125 million to successfully bring a new chemical entity to the market in 1986 compared with $54 million in 1976. Although the estimate may not be precise, it does indicate the approximate level of investment required and how that has changed over time.

Figure 7.1 summarizes the drug development process in the United States. The text below describes the steps outlined in the figure.

When basic research on human reproduction provides a lead for contraceptive development by identifying a possible point for the contraceptive intervention,

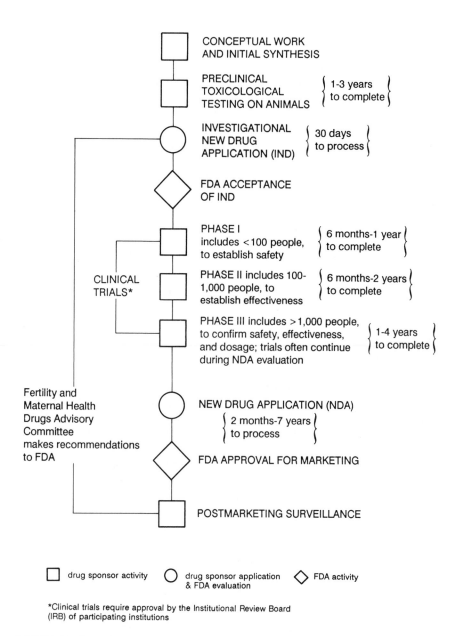

drug sponsor activity   drug sponsor application   FDA activity
& FDA evaluation

*Clinical trials require approval by the Institutional Review Board
(IRB) of participating institutions

FIGURE 7.1   The drug development process in the United States.

scientists must then determine what mechanism is best suited to take advantage of the potential point of intervention and how it can be delivered. Prototype delivery systems may then be prepared, which may be modified in light of the results of further research.

Once a drug is identified as a potential contraceptive, it must be carefully screened to establish its full range of effects. Animal studies are conducted initially to screen drugs. If the results have merit, additional animal studies and small-scale human trials follow. These early studies focus on the chemical breakdown of the drug in the body and on absorption and excretion rates. Scientists assess the drug's potency, its pharmacological effects, the onset and duration of action, chemical stability, and probable toxicity (Pasquale, 1980). At this stage the delivery system and the expected difficulty of production and formulation are also starting to be considered. Manufacturing processes would typically be designed and tested at this stage to ensure that the drug can be produced in a uniform dosage in large quantities.

Following initial synthesis and preliminary animal testing, the developer of a new contraceptive drug submits an application for claimed Investigational New Drug exemption (IND) to the Food and Drug Administration. The IND is an exemption from the statutory restriction against interstate shipment of an unapproved new drug. The IND includes information on the drug's composition, source, synthesis, and possible benefits. It also includes a detailed protocol for human testing. Human trials of the new drug may begin after a 30-day waiting period, if the FDA has not objected. If the FDA requests clarifications or more data, the drug company must respond to the FDA's satisfaction and wait another 30 days from the last response before beginning human trials.

Human clinical testing of new contraceptive drugs is divided into three phases: Phase I studies are usually conducted on a small number of volunteers and are used to determine the safe dose range, the absorption process, and possible levels of toxicity; Phase II studies provide more information about the drug's safety as well as efficacy in carefully selected subjects; and Phase III studies, which may involve several hundred or more participants, are used to establish the drug's safety and efficacy in actual clinical use. Clinical trials for new drugs take an average of five years, but they may continue for as many as 10 years (FDA, 1988).

When testing has been completed, and assuming no unacceptable problems have been discovered in the process, the developer would submit a New Drug Application (NDA) to the FDA to obtain approval to market the drug. Each NDA consists of between 2 and 15 volumes of material summarizing all the research the developer has conducted or sponsored on the drug, and 10 to 100 volumes of raw data collected during the development process (Isaacs and Holt, 1987b). The NDA for the NORPLANT® contraceptive implant, which was submitted to FDA in August 1988, contained over 19,000 pages in 53 volumes. The average review time for an NDA is two years, but it can take as long as seven years (FDA, 1988).

IUDs, which have a systemic effect because they contain copper or a hormone, are classified as drugs in the United States and must meet the premarketing requirements for drugs. The FDA approval process for new contraceptive devices, such as diaphragms and inert IUDs, is similar to that for drugs (Isaacs and Holt, 1987b), although the approval time for devices is often shorter, in part because there is usually no backlog of Premarketing Approval Applications (PMAs) for FDA review of devices (see below for more details on the regulation of devices).

The Fertility and Maternal Health Drugs Advisory Committee, a panel of outside experts who serve 4-year terms, acts as an adviser to the FDA on safety and efficacy issues related to new contraceptives and other drugs. It makes recommendations to the FDA regarding sponsors' applications to market new drugs. These recommendations, although not binding, are usually adopted by the FDA.

Once a drug is approved, the manufacturer can begin to promote it to the medical community and to the public. The FDA requires periodic reports following NDA approval and may require postmarketing studies to determine the incidence of serious adverse reactions.

A major objective of contraceptive researchers is to reduce the incidence and severity of side effects associated with systemic contraception. After more than two decades of use by millions of women, most of the risks and health benefits of oral contraceptives are known. There may, however, be adverse and beneficial effects yet to be identified that are associated with the new oral contraceptive formulations used in the past decade. (Almost all of the existing studies of oral contraceptives are based on women using high-dose pills; one hypothesis is that the newer low-dose pills will have fewer side effects, but also fewer health benefits than the high-dose pills.) Replicating this experience of widespread, long-term use of oral contraceptives in clinical trials for other methods is not yet possible. Long-term safety issues related to new systemic contraceptive methods will not be completely resolved until they have been in general use for many years.

THE REGULATION PROCESS

As a mirror of Americans' concerns and attitudes about consumer protection and the safety of drugs, Congress exerts an important influence on the FDA through legislation, hearings, and other less formal mechanisms, such as inquiries into the FDA's activities. Congress has established standards of safety and effectiveness for all drugs and medical devices marketed in the United States. These standards are contained in the Federal Food, Drug and Cosmetic Act (FFDCA) (21 U.S.C. §301 et seq. [1982 & Supp. III 1985]). The FDA is the agency responsible for the administration of the FFDCA and is empowered to promulgate regulations to aid in its enforcement.

The current FFDCA has undergone substantial legislative revisions since the original Pure Food and Drugs Act (Pub. L. No. 59-384, 34 Stat. 768 [1906]) was passed in 1906 to prevent the misbranding or adulteration of foods and drugs. In 1938, Congress added safety testing requirements to the FFDCA in response to deaths caused by a drug that had not been tested for toxicity. The 1962 amendments, drafted in response to the thalidomide tragedy, required proof of effectiveness, including "adequate and well controlled trials," prior to approval of a new drug (Pub. L. No. 87-781, 76 Stat. 780 [1962]). With the 1976 Medical Device Amendments to the FFDCA (Pub. L. No. 94-295, 21 U.S.C. §360b-360k [1976]), Congress required scientific evidence of safety and effectiveness prior to marketing new medical devices—including IUDs, many of which were not adequately regulated prior to that time. Most recently, Congress passed the Drug Price Competition and Patent Term Restoration Act of 1984 (Pub. L. No. 98-417, 98 Stat. 1598, codified principally in 21 U.S.C. §355 and 35 U.S.C. §156), which accelerates FDA approval of generic drugs and allows restoration of up to five years of patent time lost in FDA's approval of pharmaceuticals.

Congressional oversight of FDA's activities has played an important role in the approval of new contraceptives. Members of Congress have frequently responded to public concern about product safety by publicly questioning FDA officials regarding the agency's approval processes and decisions. This creates an environment of caution, in which Congress, representing public opinion, is seen to want little or no risk without significant therapeutic advantage. In 1983, for example, FDA officials were required to defend their approval of the Today contraceptive sponge (U.S. Congress, 1983). Worries about congressional reaction are also widely believed to have helped determine the nonapproval of the injectable contraceptive, Depo-Provera. The FDA receives little public credit for the timely approval of a new contraceptive, but it may suffer a serious loss of public esteem for not identifying even small risks associated with new products.

As stated above in the section on the development process, a developer of a new contraceptive does not need approval from the FDA to initiate conceptual work, laboratory testing, or preclinical research on animals. However, preclinical research is reviewed by the FDA when a contraceptive developer submits an application for FDA approval (21 C.F.R. §314.125, 314.126 [1988]). Submission of an application to the FDA (21 U.S.C. §355(i), 360j(g) [1972 & Supp. 1988]) and approval by an institutional review board (IRB), which is an oversight committee at the hospital or research institution (21 C.F.R. §312.66, 56.103 [1988]), are required before the initiation of clinical trials of a drug or device on humans, and detailed regulations apply to the design and conduct of such trials (21 C.F.R. pt. 312 [1988]).

Approval by the FDA is also needed before a new drug or device may lawfully be marketed (21 U.S.C. §355, 360e [1982]; Buday, 1987). Following FDA approval for marketing, a drug or device remains subject to numerous regulatory requirements with respect to manufacturing, labeling, and reporting of adverse experiences associated with it (21 U.S.C. §351-53, 360j(f) [1982]); 21 C.F.R. §314.80, 314.81 [1988]).

FDA's Regulation of Drugs

As described above, a party seeking to conduct clinical research (i.e., research on human subjects) on an unapproved new drug, known as the "sponsor," must submit to FDA's Center for Drug Evaluation and Research an Investigational New Drug (IND) application. The FDA requires preclinical studies before a designated new drug is tested in humans; the nature, scope, and duration of these studies depend on the nature and intended use of the drug. As the research, and therefore the use of the drug, expand in duration and/or number of subjects, the requirements for preclinical studies become more demanding. The sponsor of the research must also obtain approval from the internal review board affiliated with the institution at which the research will be conducted.

The FDA has recently revised its regulations for the investigation of new drugs with a view to reducing regulation of the early phases of human trials (U.S. Department of Health and Human Services, 1987). The FDA will seek to reduce reviews that were previously conducted solely to assess the scientific quality of the data produced by a particular protocol, but it will not reduce reviews conducted for the purpose of protecting the safety of research subjects.

It has been argued that FDA has overregulated the early phases of research and unduly inhibited scientific flexibility (a criticism intended to be met by the revised regulations), and that its protections of human subjects are unduly costly and drive research abroad. Our society is unlikely to accept less demanding protection of research subjects, and it is not known how much FDA's regulations diminish the amount of pharmaceutical research done in the United States. The United States remains the most profitable single market for most kinds of drugs, and clinical trials serve not only to develop and confirm scientific knowledge, but also to introduce a drug to physicians and the potential consumer market.

The FDA's regulation of research on contraceptives has been controversial, particularly with respect to its requirements for testing for long-term carcinogenicity in dogs and monkeys. The questions raised relate to the appropriateness of using these animals as experimental models for humans. Changes in toxicological and clinical testing requirements for contraceptive steroids implemented in 1987, however, have eliminated some of the controversial dog and monkey testing requirements.

Standards of Approval: Safety

The FFDCA requires that an application for approval of a new drug "include adequate tests by all methods reasonably applicable to show whether or not such drug is safe for use under the conditions prescribed, recommended, or suggested in the proposed labeling thereof . . ." (21 U.S.C. §355(d) [1982]). Approval is to be denied if "the results of such tests show that such drug is unsafe or do not show that such drug is safe for use under such conditions" (21 U.S.C. §355(d) [1982]). Any doubts about safety are to be resolved by denying approval.

There has been little public argument that the statutory requirements for proof of safety or that FDA's interpretation and implementation of them have been unduly demanding. Indeed, the most frequent and persistent criticism of FDA's administration of the requirements for proof of safety has been expressed in congressional hearings called to chastise the agency for being insufficiently demanding. Yet FDA's requirements for proof of safety have been a principal and highly controversial obstacle to the introduction of new contraceptive steroids.

The controversy over regulatory aspects of the safety of steroidal contraceptives focuses on two sets of issues: risk characterization and assessment and risk management (National Research Council, 1983). The first set of issues relates to the identification and quantification of the risks presented by contraceptive drugs and, in particular, the scientific appropriateness of FDA's requirements for the toxicological screening of such drugs. That set of issues is considered in this section. The second set of issues relates to the judgment of what level of risks in a new contraceptive should, for purposes of FDA approval, be acceptable in light of the benefits provided by the contraceptive. That set of issues is considered later in this chapter.

Toxicological Testing of Contraceptive Drugs   Since the introduction of the first oral contraceptives in the 1960s, the FDA's requirements for toxicological testing of proposed contraceptive drugs have been much more demanding than its requirements for the testing of other drugs. The rationale for the more severe requirements is that contraceptive drugs are intended for long-term use by millions of healthy women, most of whom have alternative contraceptive options. Given the assumed pattern of use, rigorous requirements to ensure a high degree of safety are justified. Controversy has focused, not on the FDA's objective, but rather on its strategy for achieving it.

FDA requirements for toxicological testing in animal subjects have been revised over the past 20 years. In 1968 the deputy director of the FDA's Office of New Drugs summarized the agency's requirements for toxicological testing of new contraceptive drugs (Goldenthal, 1968:14):

> We are currently requiring, as a minimum, a one-year toxicity study conducted in a rodent and the dog prior to initial clinical evaluation of [oral contraceptives] which usually consists of a three-cycle study in the human. We have also recommended, but not insisted, that a concurrent chronic study in the monkey be initiated. We have not stipulated any further toxicity requirements for continuation of these clinical pharmacology studies (Phase 2) as long as the chronic toxicity studies are ongoing. However, prior to the beginning of the large scale clinical trial (Phase 3), we have insisted that studies of up to 7 years duration in the dog and up to 10 years in the monkey be commenced. . . . The results of studies of 2 years duration in the rat, dog and monkey should be submitted in consideration for our approval of an oral contraceptive for marketing.

In the 1970s, FDA added a requirement that, prior to the initiation of large-scale Phase III clinical trials, two-year toxicity studies in rats, dogs, and monkeys be completed. Analysis of data from these animal studies can take up to two additional years, which are added to the overall time necessary for new drug development.

These requirements remained substantially unchanged until August 1987, when FDA's Advisory Committee on Fertility and Maternal Health Drugs considered the "Guidelines for the Toxicological and Clinical Assessment and Post-Registration Surveillance of Steroidal Contraceptive Drugs," which had been adopted by the World Health Organization in July 1987. The advisory committee recommended several changes in FDA's requirements, which would have made them similar both to the WHO guidelines and to the FDA's requirements for noncontraceptive drugs. In October 1987, after concluding that the required tests on animals had not been proven to have relevance to human beings, the FDA made some of the recommended changes.

The testing requirements before and after the 1987 changes are shown in Table 7.1. The testing requirements for 10-year monkey studies were completely eliminated. The 7-year testing period in beagles has been reduced to an interim testing period of 3 years, pending the release of a WHO study of the relevance of testing in beagles and its assessment by the FDA. FDA testing requirements for contraceptive steroids now conform more closely to the requirements for other drugs, with the exception of the 3-year dog studies required for contraceptive drugs.

The former requirements for 7-year beagle and 10-year monkey studies were particularly burdensome for sponsors of new contraceptives. In addition, many scientists thought the beagle studies inappropriate from a scientific point of view because of the breed's high risk of breast tumors. Together with the other chronic toxicity testing required, these tests substantially increased the cost of developing new contraceptive drugs (Djerassi, 1970). They also produced results that were interpreted as casting doubt on the safety of new contraceptives. The most dramatic case of such doubt has been Depo-Provera.

The Case of Depo-Provera   The process that resulted in the disapproval of Depo-Provera illustrates how the FDA reviews new drugs and the agency's concern for the safety of consumers. It also reveals the impact of congressional oversight as well as the impact of the legislative decision to place the burden of proof of safety on the drug sponsor.

Depo-Provera (depot-medroxyprogesterone acetate) is an injectable contraceptive administered every three months. The drug's sponsor, the Upjohn Company, sought approval of Depo-Provera for contraceptive purposes in 1967; the drug has been approved by the FDA for noncontraceptive purposes since 1960. In 1968 a 7-year study in beagles and a 10-year study in rhesus monkeys were initiated. In 1972 a second 7-year beagle study was initiated due to high mortality (attributed to pyometra) in the first study. In 1974 the FDA initially

TABLE 7.1 Comparison of Old and New Toxicological Requirements for Contraceptive Steroids

Type of Study	FDA Requirements Before 1987	1987 WHO Recommendations	1987 FDA Advisory Committee Recommendations	Current FDA Requirements Incorporating FDA and WHO Recommendations	Current FDA Requirements for Most Drugs
Acute studies	3-4 species used	1 rodent	1 rodent	3-4 species used	3-4 species used
Subchronic-chronic Studies:	Rat, dog, or monkey	2 species used	2 or 3 species used	Rodent or nonrodent; monkey as needed	Rodent or nonrodent
Phase I	90 days	flexible	2 weeks	2 weeks	2 weeks
II	1 year	flexible	4 weeks	4 weeks	4 weeks
III	2 years	1 year	6 months	6 months	6 months
NDA	—	—	1 year	1 year	1 year
Carcinogenicity studies	2 years, rat; 7 years, dog; 10 years, monkey	2 years, rat or 18 months, mouse	2 years, rat; 18 months, mouse	2 years, rat; 18 months, mouse; 3 years, dog (for interim period)	2 years, rat; 18 months, mouse

Source: Steroidal Contraceptive Toxicology Worksheet, Division of Metabolism and Endocrine Drug Products, Food and Drug Administration, October 29, 1987.

decided to approve Depo-Provera as a contraceptive for a limited patient population, but, under congressional pressure resulting from concerns about cervical cancer, the agency deferred further action.

In 1975, results from the first beagle study showed mammary tumors, including carcinomas, in treated dogs. In 1978 the FDA formally determined that Depo-Provera had not met the agency's safety standards. The FDA's reasons included the results in the first beagle study, its finding that there was no patient population in the United States that needed the drug, and its doubts about the feasibility of postmarketing surveillance in the United States to assess the risks of the drug.

Upjohn sought review of the FDA's decision by a public board of inquiry, a "science court" composed of three nongovernmental scientists appointed by the Commissioner of Food and Drugs and acceptable to Upjohn; the board for the Depo-Provera proceeding was appointed in 1981. In 1979, results of the 10-year rhesus monkey study showed endometrial cancer in two monkeys in the high-dose group. In 1982 the results of the second beagle study were reported: a high incidence of mammary nodules and carcinomas was found. The public board of inquiry, after holding hearings and receiving reports from its own consultants, issued its report on October 17, 1984. It upheld the denial of approval of the contraceptive indication for Depo-Provera in the United States.

The board concluded that the second beagle study was well designed and well conducted, that it showed a dose-response relationship, and that in the study the observed carcinogenic effects were attributable to Depo-Provera. It also concluded that the monkey study was poorly designed and conducted; that it did not show a dose-response relationship; but that uterine carcinomas in rhesus monkeys are unexpected and not known to occur spontaneously; and, therefore, that there was reason to assume that the carcinomas were related to the drug. The board concluded that, until proven otherwise, the endometrial carcinomas in the monkeys should be viewed as related to Depo-Provera. This result was, in effect, an allocation of a burden of proof: in the face of a currently unexplainable adverse result, the burden is on the sponsor of the drug to show to the satisfaction of qualified scientists that a given result is not related to the drug in question, rather than on the regulatory agency to show that a result is related to the drug. This allocation of the burden is required by the FFDCA.

Richard and Lasagna (1987) have analyzed how differences in drug regulatory philosophy and clinical requirements in the United States and the United Kingdom resulted in the approval of Depo-Provera for contraceptive purposes in the United Kingdom but not in the United States. The U.S. public board of inquiry and the U.K. review panel both reviewed the available scientific data, but their assessments and recommendations were quite different. In Great Britain, the panel reviewing Depo-Provera found that the evidence did not show that it was unsafe and therefore approved it. The U.S. board of inquiry found that the available evidence did not prove that Depo-Provera was safe, however, and therefore did not recommend approval. The difference in outcomes seems to have resulted not from scientific differences, but from the policy differences (burden of proof) in the laws of the two countries.

Upjohn appealed the board's decision to the Commissioner of Food and Drugs; subsequently, it sought to reopen the administrative record to permit introduction of additional data. When that request was denied, Upjohn withdrew its appeal and its supplemental application for approval of the contraceptive indication pending the completion of additional studies. As of this writing, Upjohn representatives say the company has no plans to resubmit its application for approval of Depo-Provera for contraceptive purposes in the United States.

The Appropriateness of Current Safety Requirements for Contraceptive Drugs
The FDA's requirements for tests of contraceptive drugs in beagles and monkeys reflect a demand for proof of safety that applies to all drugs but is, perhaps, uniquely burdensome to sponsors of contraceptives. The statutory requirement for "*adequate* tests by *all* methods reasonably applicable to show whether or not [the] drug is safe" (emphasis added) and the provision that approval shall be denied if "such tests . . . do not show that [the] drug is safe . . . ." (21 U.S.C. §355(d) [1982]) reflect an apparent congressional view that the safety of a drug can be conclusively determined before it is approved. Such a view is scientifically incorrect.

The clinical testing of a drug in a few thousand human subjects ordinarily can identify the drug's relatively common adverse effects, but it cannot identify the relatively uncommon effects. Those will appear and be recognized only after approval, when the population of patients exposed to the drug increases from a few thousand to tens or hundreds of thousands or even millions. Moreover, chronic adverse effects generally cannot be identified at all from human studies prior to approval; extrapolations must be made from studies in animals. Thus, at the time the FDA decides whether or not to approve a drug, the drug's complete profile of adverse effects is not available. Consequently, a decision to approve necessarily involves some risk of unknown adverse effects that will appear and be linked to the drug later. The subsequent identification of adverse effects at times leads to a reinterpretation of data from the clinical trials, which is followed by criticism of the FDA for not having recognized as drug-related adverse effects that, prior to approval, were viewed by both the sponsor and the agency as not drug-related. Thus, approval of a drug puts the FDA at institutional risk.

The size of the risk that serious adverse effects will be discovered after approval depends on several factors, including the size of the anticipated patient population, the duration of anticipated use by individual patients, the relevant medical characteristics of those patients, and the circumstances of use. With some classes of drugs, the FDA is reasonably comfortable running this risk. With others, the agency is sufficiently uncomfortable that it conditions approval on agreement by drug developers to conduct postapproval epidemiological studies of adverse events associated with the approved drugs.

With or without such a study, the manufacturer of an approved drug has a legal obligation to inform FDA of possible drug-related adverse reactions that are not already identified in the official labeling for the drug or that appear to be occurring with greater frequency or greater severity than is suggested in the labeling (see generally 21 C.F.R. §314.80 [1988]). Manufacturers may learn of such reactions from physicians, patients, the worldwide medical literature, or products liability claims. FDA does not consider such spontaneous reports a substitute for the data derivable from controlled trials; rather, the spontaneous reports are signals that effects are occurring that may warrant detailed attention.

Virtually any approved contraceptive drug has a potential patient population of millions, and patients may use the drug continuously over a period of years. The principal risk of concern for several contraceptives—cancer—is a chronic risk, with a latency period of possibly 10 to 40 years. To obtain conclusive data on the human carcinogenicity of a contraceptive drug thus might require that very large numbers of users be exposed to the drug over a very long period of time. If a drug demonstrably offers unique dramatic benefits—if, for example, it literally saves lives or cures a severely disabling disease and has no substitute—it is fairly easy to conclude that this risk of the unknown is worth taking. Is such a risk worth taking, however, in the case of a contraceptive drug, even one with a unique method of administration that offers unique convenience? The answer to that question depends on how the FDA weighs benefits and risks in evaluating a drug for approval. A discussion of that calculation follows our consideration of FDA procedures for reviewing the effectiveness of a new contraceptive drug.

Standards of Approval: Effectiveness

The 1962 amendments to the FFDCA expressly required, for the first time, that new drugs be shown to be effective (as well as safe) prior to their approval by the FDA (Pub. L. No. 87-781, 76 Stat. 780 [1962]). The statute requires, as a precondition for approval of a new drug, "substantial evidence that the drug will have the effect it purports or is represented to have under the conditions of use prescribed, recommended, or suggested in the proposed labeling thereof . . . ." (21 U.S.C. §355(d) [1982]). The FDA has interpreted the statute as requiring at least two clinical studies to establish substantial evidence of effectiveness (21 C.F.R. §314.125, 314.126 [1988]).

The FDA's implementation of the statute and regulations during the last two decades has been the subject of lengthy public dispute. Some analysts argue that the requirements have merely introduced to the field of pharmaceutical research standards of scientific quality well established in other fields; that the requirements protect the public from ineffective drugs and lead to the generation of data that are useful as prescription guidelines once a drug is approved; and that the requirements are necessary because of the difficulty in removing from the market an approved drug that is later found to be ineffective. Others contend that the FDA's demands for scientific proof have driven up the cost of drug research and development, retarded drug innovation, delayed the introduction of important new drugs, and deprived the American public of some useful drugs altogether. The public policy debate about the costs and benefits of FDA requirements for proof of effectiveness relates to new drugs generally, not to contraceptives in particular. In fact, contraceptive effectiveness has been relatively easy to establish and, consequently, the general requirements for proof of effectiveness have not adversely affected contraceptive innovation in any distinctive way. Issues have arisen regarding the minimal effective dose of some contraceptive drugs, however, and regulatory approval of reduced doses of some products in the United States has lagged behind similar approvals in Europe.

There is an important distinction between contraceptive effectiveness in a controlled clinical study and contraceptive effectiveness in general use. The effectiveness of a contraceptive in a controlled clinical trial may be significantly higher than effectiveness in actual use in the general population over an extended period. Moreover, different segments of a population may have different views on the relative importance of effectiveness versus other factors, such as the incidence of minor acute side effects, risk of chronic illness, or cost.

The Risk-Benefit Trade-off All active drugs cause adverse effects in some users. If safety were understood as the total absence of adverse effects, then no drug could be called "safe." Safety of a drug is conceived as a favorable ratio of benefits to risks for the population of users of the drug as a whole. That ratio is determined by the FDA when considering whether to approve a drug. In the case of a prescription drug to be used by an individual, an individualized ratio is determined, in light of the available knowledge about the drug and about the patient, by the patient's physician in consultation with the patient. (In theory, in the case of an over-the-counter drug, the same type of assessment should be made by the patient or by the person administering the drug, guided by the directions for use in the drug's labeling.)

When considering whether to approve a drug, the FDA evaluates its medical benefits and risks against a specific health condition or illness. The benefits considered in evaluating a particular drug are, generally, its benefits to the individuals or groups who would use it. In some cases, for example vaccines, the FDA also gives weight to clear and direct benefits to public health, including the health of persons who would not use the drug. The agency does not consider other kinds of benefits, such as economic benefits. If contraceptives have benefits that are external to individual users and that do not directly benefit the public health, an amendment to the FFDCA by Congress would be necessary before the FDA could consider them.

The benefits that FDA considers are benefits to patients in the United States. The agency can approve the export from the United States of a drug that has not been approved for marketing in the United States, but, in deciding whether to approve a drug for marketing in this country, under the law the agency may not consider the effects of its decision in other countries. Nonetheless, the FDA's decisions with respect to contraceptives may have an important impact on the provision of family planning services in less developed countries. These countries, for example, may not allow the import of drugs not approved by the FDA, and the Agency for International Development's practice is to provide only contraceptive commodities that are approved by FDA to developing country health and family planning programs.

In general, the value of the specific medical benefits provided by a drug (e.g., lowering blood pressure, reducing retention of fluids, shrinking tumors) is a matter of technical medical judgment; the same is true of risks. The value of some medical benefits, however, transcends a merely professional judgment: physicians and biological scientists have difficulty assessing the value of avoiding an unwanted pregnancy or of the nonmedical aspects of a particular means of contraception, because the criteria are less clear or are difficult to measure. But few disagree that the ability to determine the number and spacing of one's children can be an important influence on people's health and economic well-being. In weighing the benefits and risks of contraceptive drugs, therefore, the FDA's physicians and scientists engage in a task that is at least potentially different from the one they perform in evaluating other kinds of drugs.

Of course, decisions about contraceptives may, in some circumstances, present no special difficulty. If a proposed new drug has *no* advantages in any respect when compared with an already approved drug but presents additional risks, then a decision to deny its approval is easily reached. Similarly, if a new contraceptive has modest advantages compared with previously approved drugs but also causes serious side effects, the ratio of benefits to risks is clearly unfavorable.

The proper outcome is less clear, however, when, for example, the new drug has unique benefits, an acceptable acute toxicity, but chronic toxicity that is unknown or is known only not to be strong. In these circumstances, there is room for debate about the appropriate benefit-risk standard for approval. On one hand it might be argued, for example, that low (but actual) risks of cancer or other chronic diseases might rationally be accepted by a woman for whom effective contraception (or effective contraception by a particular mode) is of very great present value, perhaps because other contraceptive methods are not likely to be completely effective over the long term or are simply unacceptable for cultural, religious, or other reasons and pregnancy itself could present a grave medical risk. Moreover, because of the risks associated with pregnancy, labor, and delivery, use of less effective contraceptives may have more risk for some women. On the other hand it might be argued that drugs that present risks of serious chronic toxicity can be considered safe only when they provide lifesaving benefits, and that a contraceptive that is a carcinogen in animals should not be approved unless it is scientifically established that the drug's carcinogenicity in animals is irrelevant to its effects in humans. A range of intermediate positions is also possible.

The FDA's current view on approval of new contraceptives was expressed by Commissioner Arthur Hull Hayes, Jr., M.D., at a congressional hearing called in 1983 to review the agency's approval of the Today contraceptive sponge (U.S. Congress, 1983:130):

> It is important to recognize that this new contraceptive product, like all contraceptive products, will be used primarily by healthy people. Moreover, alternative methods of contraception are available that are very safe—although some methods . . . are not without some risk—and have a very substantial use experience. Because of this, a new contraceptive such as the sponge must meet a very high standard of safety. While significant risks may be acceptable for some drugs in light of the benefit to be derived by the sick patient, the contraceptive sponge must not present a significant risk to the user.

To change the FDA's standard for the minimum acceptable benefit-risk ratio of new contraceptives would require action by Congress—either new legislation specifically directing the agency to apply a different standard or directives to that effect from the relevant congressional committees. At the present time, there is no indication that any such action to change the FDA's policy is likely to be forthcoming.

The FDA has recognized that values and preferences of patients should play a role in the selection of a contraceptive. To facilitate informed participation by patients in the process of selection, the agency has required manufacturers of contraceptives to provide patient package inserts with their products. These inserts present, in lay language, the principal information on method of use, effectiveness, and safety relevant to the decision. (Consumers are left on their own to compare the costs of alternative products.)

Issues surrounding the evaluation of benefits and risks of a new contraceptive become more complicated when consideration is extended to cases in which users are incapable of making a well-informed assessment of benefits and risks or in which they are entirely incompetent and the decision is made by a private or public provider of care (whose interests may, in some respects, diverge from those of the user). In deciding whether a contraceptive drug presenting some chronic risks should be approved for marketing to the general population, most of whom can, with medical advice, make a well-informed decision, the weight the FDA should give to the special vulnerabilities of particular groups within the population has been a particular concern. This was and remains an element in the debate about the reasonableness of the FDA's disapproval of Depo-Provera.

No law, judicial decision, or agency policy of general applicability tells the FDA how to weigh the effects of a drug on users who do not know how to use it properly or whose views with respect to its use cannot be ascertained or will not be taken into account when individual prescribing decisions are made. The FDA makes such decisions on an ad hoc basis. In exercising its discretion to decide what risks of a contraceptive are acceptable in light of its benefits, the agency will be influenced, to varying degrees, by the various constituencies that are interested in the question: the scientific community, the family planning community, congressional committee and subcommittee chairs, women's organizations, contraceptive manufacturers, consumer groups, public interest groups, and editorial writers. There appears to be little likelihood that the FDA will become more lenient toward risks in the foreseeable future.

Patent Life and Profitability Developers of new contraceptives protect their investment in research and development by securing patents from the Patent and Trademark Office in the U.S. Department of Commerce. Patents grant inventors 17-year exclusive rights to manufacture and sell their products. In theory, the 17-year patent duration, which generally begins long before FDA review, allows developers to recoup their investment in R&D by temporarily protecting their products from competitors who would otherwise be able to offer the same product at a lower price. The Federal Food, Drug, and Cosmetic Act also provides certain periods of nonpatent marketing exclusivity, which can extend to more than five years.

Levin (1986, 1988), Griliches et al. (1987), and Mansfield (1986) have examined the value of patents in technological innovation and inventive activity and how patentability influences corporate decisions to pursue new product development. Although information is not available on contraceptive products per se, the results of these and other studies show that patents are especially valuable in the pharmaceutical industry. However, FDA requirements for data on a product's safety and effectiveness and the length of time needed for FDA review have contributed to a reduction in the length of time from the date of FDA approval until the date of patent expiration (the effective patent life) of new products. This reduction makes investment in R&D less attractive than it would be if patent life began when a product was approved for marketing by the FDA, for example.

Grabowski and Vernon (1983) have examined the effect on profitability of changes in effective patent life, as well as different degrees of product substitution, and changing R&D costs associated with shorter regulatory approval times. The results of their study indicate that about two-thirds of the new chemical entities introduced during the 1970–1976 period had not recovered their full R&D costs. Although the median return on drug R&D investment was low, a small number of products earned several times the average R&D costs. Grabowski and Vernon conclude that pharmaceutical companies are heavily dependent on developing a small number of highly successful products that will dominate a particular therapeutic market to cover total R&D investments.

During the past two decades, there has been a steady decline in the mean effective patent life for New Chemical Entities (NCEs) introduced in the United States—from 14.4 years in 1967 to 7.9 years in 1984 (Eisman and Wardell, 1981; Kaitin and Trimble, 1987). This decline in effective patent life directly correlates with an increase in the mean number of years from IND submission to NDA approval. Between 1964 and 1984, the mean duration of the regulatory phase for U.S.-originated NCEs increased from 4.5 years to 9.5 years (Mattison et al.,

1988). The total time for self-originated NCEs owned by U.S. firms, including the preclinical and regulatory phases, has increased from less than 7 years in 1964 to more than 16 years in 1984. These figures, however, include all NCEs; because of the more extensive animal testing requirements for new contraceptive steroids before 1987 (e.g., 10-year monkey studies and 7-year beagle studies), the average total development time of new contraceptive drugs is likely to have been much longer. (It was not possible to obtain data on total development time from the manufacturers of contraceptive NCEs.)

The Drug Price Competition and Patent Term Restoration Act of 1984 (the 1984 DPC-PTR Act) was enacted to help alleviate problems of short effective patent life for drugs and medical devices. The 1984 act is the most important drug legislation since the 1962 amendments to the FFDCA (Kaitin and Trimble, 1987). In an attempt to reduce the cost of drugs through the encouragement of competition, the act streamlined the requirements for FDA approval of generic drugs. A significant provision of the act restores up to five years to patent life for patent time lost during the drug development and approval process. Given the five-year increase in the mean duration of the regulatory phase between 1964 and 1984 (Mattison et al., 1988), the restoration of up to five years of patent life is a potentially significant incentive for innovation by the pharmaceutical industry. The 1984 DPC-PTR Act also provides varying time periods (up to five years plus the FDA's review time) of market exclusivity to new drugs, during which time the FDA will not approve a substitute or alternative for the product.

The impact of the 1984 DPC-PTR Act on effective patent life has yet to be determined. A study by the Center for Drug Development at Tufts University (Kaitin and Trimble, 1987) indicates that during the first two years of its implementation, the 1984 act has favored generic drug firms over the companies developing new drugs. This result is to be expected, as the benefits of patent life restoration to developers of new drugs will not be fully evident until drugs currently being developed are eligible for the full five years of patent extension.

Grabowski and Vernon (1983) argue that reductions in the early R&D costs and in delays associated with regulation will have a greater impact on the economic incentives to undertake innovative research than comparable gains in patent life added at the end of the market exclusivity period. They point out, however, that it is easier to change patent protection policy by legislative action than it is to shorten regulatory delays and eliminate cost inefficiencies. Nevertheless, they conclude that regulatory reform should continue to be a high priority. Reductions in effective R&D cost could be achieved by changes in tax policy or governmental subsidization of research.

FDA's Regulation of Medical Devices

Contraceptives such as intrauterine devices, diaphragms, and condoms are regulated as medical devices by the FDA's Center for Devices and Radiological

Health. Although the regulatory forms and terminology applicable to devices differ from those applicable to drugs, and the specific issues of safety vary between drugs and devices (as they do, of course, among drugs and among devices), substantially similar general requirements for the demonstration of safety and effectiveness and a favorable ratio of benefits to risks apply to both categories of products.

The system for regulation of medical devices is more complex than that for regulation of drugs, and a full exposition is beyond the scope of this chapter (see Munsey and Samuel, 1984). A brief summary is sufficient, however, for an understanding of how the FDA regulates contraceptive devices.

Under the 1976 medical device amendments to the FFDCA, all categories of devices are classified by the FDA into one of three classes. Class I devices, the simplest and the least regulated, are subject to the statute's general controls: prohibitions of adulteration and misbranding; registration of manufacturers and listing of specific devices in submissions to the FDA; vulnerability to being banned if they are deceptive or present an unreasonable and substantial risk of illness or injury; vulnerability to an order by the FDA requiring notification to health professionals and others of a risk to the public health or an order by the FDA requiring repair, replacement, or refund; record-keeping and reporting obligations; vulnerability to an order by the FDA restricting the distribution of the device; and good manufacturing practice requirements. Facilities in which any device is manufactured, processed, packed, or held in the course of interstate commerce are subject to inspection by the FDA. There are no contraceptive devices categorized as Class I; examples of Class I devices include adhesive bandages and toothbrushes.

Class II devices are subject to all the general controls that apply to Class I devices and are also, in theory, subject to performance standards developed or adopted by the FDA. Condoms and diaphragms are examples of Class II devices. In principle, Class II devices are ones for which the general controls "are insufficient to provide reasonable assurance of the safety and effectiveness of the device [and] for which there is sufficient information to establish a performance standard to provide such assurance. . . ." (21 U.S.C. §360c(a)(1)(B) (1972 and Supp. 1989). Thus far, however, the FDA has not established any performance standards, and there is no prospect that it will. This aspect of the statute has simply proven unworkable. The FDA's position is that, for Class II devices, the general controls, together with the FDA's general rulemaking authority, compliance programs, and enforcement actions provide adequate assurance of safety and effectiveness. Both Class I and Class II devices may be introduced into commercial distribution without prior approval by the FDA.

Class III devices are subject to all the general controls that apply to Class I and Class II devices and are also subject to specific device-by-device premarketing approval by the FDA. Examples of Class III devices include tubal occlusion plugs, sterilization clips, and inert IUDs. The factors that determine whether a device will be classified as Class III are (a) there is insufficient information to determine that the general controls are sufficient to provide reasonable assurance of safety and effectiveness, (b) there is insufficient information for establishment of a performance standard to provide that assurance, and (c) the device is represented for a use in supporting or sustaining human life or for a use of substantial importance in preventing impairment of human health, or it presents a potential unreasonable risk of illness or injury. Any new device is automatically classified as Class III unless it is reclassified as Class I or Class II or is substantially equivalent to one of two types of devices described below.

There are three principal routes to the marketplace for a new contraceptive device. The first route is through premarketing approval and is the standard route intended by Congress. The second route, which has emerged as by far the most common route, is called a "section 510(k) notice." Through this procedure, the manufacturer of a new device demonstrates to the FDA that, with respect to all aspects of performance that relate to safety or effectiveness, the new device is substantially equivalent to (or better than) a functionally similar device marketed prior to the enactment of the medical device amendments (May 28, 1976) or to some other device that has been classified as Class I or Class II. The demonstration is made in a notice to the FDA in which the manufacturer supports a claim of substantial equivalence to a specified device. If the FDA does not object to the claim within 90 days, the manufacturer may market the new device. The FDA, of course, may later take enforcement action against the device on the ground that it is not substantially equivalent as claimed by the manufacturer, but such action by the agency is most unlikely. The §510(k) notice was not contemplated by Congress in 1976 as a potentially significant route to the market for new devices.

The third route to the market for a new device is for its manufacturer to obtain from the FDA, by petition, a reclassification (from Class III to Class II or to Class I) of the category of devices to which the new device belongs. This route is in most respects as burdensome as premarketing approval, and it has been used infrequently.

Condoms and diaphragms are currently classified as Class II; inert IUDs and tubal occlusion devices for sterilization are classified in Class III (21 C.F.R. §884.5300, 884.5310, 884.5350, 884.5360, and 884.5380 [1988]). Prior to the 1976 medical device amendments, inert IUDs (e.g., Dalkon shield, Lippes loop), diaphragms, condoms, and tubal occlusion devices were subject to the FFDCA but were not subject to premarketing approval by the FDA. Many of these products were allowed to stay on the market after 1976 under grandfather provisions of the medical device amendments.

Developers of new contraceptive devices must submit an Investigational Device Exemption (IDE) to the FDA (21 U.S.C. §360j(q) [1982]). This application is comparable to the IND for investigational new drugs and permits the developer to test the new device in human populations, provided that testing will be supervised by an institutional review board, that appropriate informed consent will be obtained, and that certain records and reports will be maintained.

The next stage in the FDA approval process for Class III contraceptive devices is the Premarket Approval Application (PMA), which is comparable to an NDA for a new drug (21 U.S.C. §360e [1982]). Once the PMA is received by the FDA, the agency attempts to respond to the applicant within six months. The product must be evaluated by an obstetrics and gynecology advisory panel that makes recommendations to the FDA regarding the approval of the device.

For a new device that is claimed to be equivalent in safety and effectiveness to a pre-1976 device already on the market (e.g., condoms and diaphragms) and that FDA has classified as Class I or II (i.e., not requiring premarketing approval), the manufacturer must submit to the FDA a notice demonstrating equivalency to the already marketed product but does not have to submit a PMA (21 U.S.C. §360(k) [1982]). The FDA review period for such applications is 90 days, but the actual review period may be longer due to incomplete applications from the manufacturer and requests for clarifications and additional evidence by the FDA.

Impediments to FDA Approval

A number of factors may cause delay in the approval of new drugs and devices. A 1980 study by the General Accounting Office (GAO) found the following problems: (1) FDA guidelines were imprecise; (2) reviewers of NDAs changed; (3) scientific and professional disagreements between the FDA and the industry were slow to be resolved; (4) the FDA's feedback to industry about deficiencies was slow; (5) chemistry and manufacturing control reviews were especially slow; and (6) the industry submitted incomplete NDAs. In recent years, however, the FDA has made significant efforts to eliminate or reduce some of these problems.

For contraceptive products approved between 1962 and 1987, it is possible to calculate the mean duration between the date an NDA was received by the FDA and the date it was approved for marketing. For oral contraceptives (96 different formulations), the average time was 19 months; for intrauterine devices (5 products), it was 26 months; for vaginal contraceptive products (3 products), it was 13 months (FDA, 1988). The recent changes by the FDA in toxicological testing requirements for new contraceptive steroidal drugs may help to speed up the approval process for new contraceptive drugs by reducing the amount of data the FDA must review. It should be mentioned, however, that the NDA review period is only a small fraction of the total time necessary to develop and obtain approval of a new contraceptive drug or device.

Although claims have been made that the FDA is making progress in speeding the approval process, analysis of NDA approval trends for contraceptives shows mixed results. For example, of oral contraceptive NDA applications received in the 1960s (36 formulations), the average time to approval was 27 months; of oral contraceptive NDA applications received in the 1970s (37 formulations), the average time to approval had dropped to only 12 months. However, of oral contraceptive NDA applications received in the 1980s (23 formulations), the average time to approval had risen to over 16 months.

Postmarketing Surveillance

Some risk is inevitable with all contraceptives, whether it is a health risk or the risk of pregnancy because of contraceptive failure. It is impossible to know what the long-term risks or benefits of a new contraceptive will be until many years after the product has been in use and many thousands of person-years of use have accumulated. Increases in scientific knowledge of risks and benefits does not come in steady increments. The risks of oral contraceptives, for example, were known before many of their beneficial health effects were discovered.

At present, postmarketing surveillance systems for contraceptive products are not adequate. No long-term epidemiological studies of the health risks and benefits of the new oral contraceptive formulations that have been introduced during the past two decades in the United States are under way. To evaluate the impact of oral contraceptives on diseases such as breast cancer, scientists must rely on data on higher-dose contraceptives, some brands of which have been taken off the market. In the past, consumers have carried the bulk of the burden of inadequate or nonexistent postmarketing surveillance in the form of higher prices for products or in the form of excessive injuries.

Although the need for more postmarketing surveillance is clear, there are a number of obstacles to a successful surveillance system. These include the problems of confidentiality of medical records, development of appropriate data bases and methodologies, and financing these often very costly studies. Furthermore, there is often a long lag time between the actual experience of users and the final results of the analysis of postmarketing surveillance studies. Discussion of the details of this complex topic is beyond the scope of this report. As noted above, however, the assumption is that contraceptives are used for long periods of time by millions of healthy people and that there is a long latency period for the potentially most important and most worrisome risks. Thus, although we do not wish to make detailed recommendations on improvements in postmarketing surveillance systems, we believe such improvements are necessary.

CONTRACEPTIVE REGULATION:
AN INTERNATIONAL PERSPECTIVE

Like the FDA, national drug regulatory agencies in other countries have requirements for the approval of contraceptives that exceed the requirements for other drugs (Rowe, 1983). These additional requirements exist because (1) prevention of unwanted pregnancy is not considered to be a curative therapy or prophylaxis; (2) recipients of contraceptive drugs are still exposed to the risk of pregnancy because no contraceptive is 100 percent effective; and (3) contraceptive drugs are taken for longer periods than most other drugs.

Regulatory standards for drugs and medical devices vary among countries with respect to: (1) product development, (2) effectiveness, (3) safety, (4) packaging and quality control, (5) instructions for use, (6) consumer protection, (7) product availability, and (8) pricing (Cook et al., 1982). Although differences among countries in regulatory requirements are probably related to international differences in contraceptive development efforts, broader social and economic factors play a much more important role in determining the extent to which contraceptive development takes place in particular countries.

A 1980 study by the General Accounting Office identified several key differences in the regulatory processes in the Netherlands, Norway, Sweden, the United Kingdom, and Canada compared with the United States (GAO, 1980). The GAO concluded that the regulatory processes in these countries were generally faster and more flexible. Among the key differences between the countries studied and the United States were: (1) greater use of expert committees, (2) greater acceptance of foreign data, (3) less politicizing of the drug approval process, and (4) greater cooperation between regulators and industry (GAO, 1980; National Academy of Engineering, 1983).

The mean number of months from the NDA application for marketing a new drug to the date when regulatory approval was granted varied widely among the countries: the United Kingdom, 5 months; Canada, 16 months; Norway, 17 months; the United States, 23 months; and Sweden, 28 months (GAO, 1980). It should be pointed out, however, that the period from the filing of the NDA to the date of approval is only a very short segment of the total time required for new drug development. Furthermore, these figures include applications with very minor changes or modifications that are included as NDAs.

Regulation in Europe

European pharmaceutical firms generally follow the European Economic Community (EEC) directives for new drug applications when submitting new contraceptives for approval in Western Europe. Following approval in one EEC country, a drug company may expect expeditious reviews in other EEC countries. Nevertheless, simultaneous submissions to several countries are frequently made to circumvent possible delays in the review procedure in the first country. This approach is viewed by the drug industry as superior to the establishment of a complex supranational European regulatory agency.

Some European drug industry experts view the FDA's revision of its toxicological and clinical testing requirements for new contraceptive steroids as a very positive development. Moreover, although a 3-year beagle study is still required by the FDA and none is required by EEC countries, the FDA has indicated that this requirement will be reviewed in light of the findings of a study currently being completed. Although toxicological requirements for testing new contraceptive steroids in Europe and the United States are now much more similar than they have been, European drug companies are still concerned about such issues as whether approval will be granted on the basis of European clinical data only, the FDA's monitoring requirements for clinical studies conducted outside the United States, and FDA requirements for availability of raw data on the subjects of clinical research.

The lack of price control makes the United States an attractive country for the introduction of new contraceptive products. In Europe, the prices of contraceptives are normally controlled by governments, and companies claim that low profit margins barely allow recovery of R&D costs. Because of the size of the U.S. market, as well as its potential for higher profits than Europe, regulatory changes in the United States may affect contraceptive development activities in Europe as well as in the United States.

The United States is not the only country that has seen a decline in the effective patent life of contraceptives and other pharmaceuticals. No patent life restoration legislation exists in Europe. However, the United States and the EEC both have legislation that protects the exclusive marketing rights of a pharmaceutical company that submits a file for regulatory approval, regardless of the patent situation. In Europe, files of new products remain inaccessible (and therefore cannot be used by competitors to gain marketing approval for generic copies) for up to 10 years from the time the first EEC country approval has been granted; in the United States the FFDCA grants up to 5 years of exclusive marketing rights from the time of FDA approval. Formal patent life in the United States is 17 years, while in Europe it is 20 years.

Regulation in Developing Countries

Because of limited resources and limited expertise, many developing countries base their regulatory decisions on the status of drugs or devices in the developed countries where they are produced or marketed. For example, the Zimbabwean government, through its Drugs Control Council, will not approve any drug that is not approved for public use in its country of origin (Mutambirwa, 1988). A number of developing countries, such as Bangladesh and Nepal, do not rely on the status of a product in the exporting country; in those countries, the ministries of health oversee the approval of new drugs and medical devices (including contraceptives). A special medical review panel is often established to perform this function (Cook et al., 1982).

A few developing countries have well-established drug registration agencies, whose principal concern is the introduction and sale of new drugs (Rowe, 1983). In those countries, import and export restrictions, tariffs, laws governing manufacturing, and corporate and university research could have an important effect on the development and introduction of new products. This is the case in India, where research on new contraceptives is well advanced. The current government of India has made several changes in the domestic regulatory environment that are encouraging greater growth and development of a private pharmaceutical industry (e.g., exempting various pharmaceutical products from licensing requirements; easing of licensing requirements for additional capacity; and relaxing controls over foreign collaboration). The revised governmental policies have encouraged the private sector to begin to produce contraceptives. In 1987, the production of Copper T200 IUDs was initiated by both the public and the private sectors. The government is also encouraging private-sector involvement in the production of oral contraceptives and has recently removed price controls for oral contraceptives.

The World Health Organization's Role

In addition to its efforts to develop new contraceptives, the World Health Organization plays a role in the regulation of contraceptives. WHO works with governmental agencies, pharmaceutical companies, and nonprofit research organizations on the international harmonization of drug regulations; on updating official requirements for preclinical and clinical assessments of new fertility regulating agents; on postmarketing surveillance of contraceptives; and on the provision of advice and assistance, especially to developing countries, on the safety and efficacy of contraceptives.

In recent years there has been increasing international cooperation among drug regulatory agencies in different countries, as well as between the international pharmaceutical firms and regulatory agencies (Lasagna and Werko, 1986). The World Health Organization has helped bring about more international uniformity in the regulation and control of pharmaceutical drugs and other medical products.

As of the early 1980s, 55 developing countries were participating in WHO's "Certification on the Quality of Pharmaceutical Products Moving in International Commerce Scheme" (Rowe, 1983). This program provides information to importing countries about whether a given product has been authorized to be placed on the market in the exporting country and, if it has not been authorized, on the reasons why.

There has been some discussion about establishing uniform international drug regulations, but to date little interest in this has been shown by pharmaceutical companies or national drug regulatory agencies (Rowe, 1983). Since many countries do not have strong drug regulatory agencies and since the regulatory requirements and procedures of other countries vary widely, some have proposed that WHO regulate at least some products. In 1982, for example, representatives from the International Planned Parenthood Federation suggested that WHO become "an international drug regulatory mechanism for contraceptives" (WHO, 1984:1). This idea was reiterated at the International Symposium on Research on the Regulation of Human Fertility in 1983. In fact, a review was undertaken by WHO to explore "the role WHO might play, the feasibility and the additional cost of becoming an international drug regulatory agency for contraceptives" (WHO, 1984:1). WHO concluded that it did not have a mandate from its member states to establish itself as a regulatory authority. Whether or not WHO assumes formal regulatory responsibilities, increasing the role it plays internationally in providing advice, assistance, and information on the safety, effectiveness, and regulatory status of new contraceptive drugs and devices would probably help to facilitate international decisions regarding the approval of new contraceptive products.

RECOMMENDATIONS

The committee does not wish to reduce the safety requirements applicable to contraceptives. Instead, our objective is to add new criteria to the evaluation of safety to make it more meaningful and more specific to different groups of potential users.

The committee recommends that the FDA increases the weight it assigns to contraceptive effectiveness and convenience of use. The effect of such a change is that a benefit-risk ratio that currently would be viewed as inadequate to support approval might be viewed as adequate. Such an approval should be subject to certain conditions intended to ensure that the approval will increase, rather than decrease, the long-term health of users of the new contraceptive.

First, whenever appropriate such a contraceptive should be indicated only for a well-defined population that, in fact, is not adequately served by other contraceptives. Second, both the physician labeling (in professional language) and patient labeling (in lay terms) of the contraceptive should discuss the basis for the FDA's benefit-risk assessment and any and all significant risks to health presented by the contraceptive. The labeling should also suggest that a decision on whether or not to use the contraceptive should take into account the full array of risks presented by the contraceptive, the importance of avoiding pregnancy for health or other reasons, the effectiveness of this particular contraceptive, and the relative benefits and risks of other methods. The point of the labeling is that the patient, with advice from the physician, should make an informed choice. Third, approval should be followed by long-term studies of actual effectiveness in use and of adverse effects and any health benefits from use.

The committee does not consider an increase in the weight ascribed to contraceptive effectiveness and convenience to be a major change in the FDA's regulation of contraceptives or a departure from the public policy that the FDA applies with respect to other drugs. Rather, we view it as an effort to make the FDA's regulation of contraceptive drugs and devices more similar to its regulation of other drugs and devices. The committee does not believe that the proposed change would justify, or would bring about, any reduction in public confidence in the effectiveness or safety of contraceptive products. The purpose of the change is to provide new contraceptives for particular groups in the population who are not adequately served by the current array of contraceptive products. For these subpopulations, we wish to encourage the FDA to consider new contraceptives that are effective and that—in light of their effectiveness and other qualities, and given the relative advantages and disadvantages of other contraceptive options and the needs of individual users—have a risk profile that is acceptable socially, medically, and to the value systems of users. If these limitations are adhered to, and if proper information is provided to physicians and patients, this proposed change (together with the other changes proposed by the committee) should have no effect on the rules of products liability that should otherwise be applicable to contraceptive products (see Chapter 8).

Contraceptive effectiveness helps women not only avoid unwanted pregnancy, but also avoid the medical risks that, for some women, would be associated with pregnancy and childbirth. Convenience is crucial to acceptability and actual use and therefore to effectiveness of use in a nonclinical setting. More generally, control of fertility itself is of very great value to many women and men; that value, even though unquantifiable, should be recognized in benefit-risk evaluations.

The FDA should also be prepared to approve, in some circumstances, a new contraceptive drug or device that presents a risk if it is shown that the new contraceptive offers a safety advantage for an identifiable group of users when compared with that group's current actual contraceptive practice (including nonuse). That is, in some circumstances a new contraceptive may, for some users, be safer than currently used contraceptives, even though the new product presents a risk that is nontrivial, and even though equally or more safe contraceptives are available but are not used by that group. In such circumstances, denial of approval of the new product on the ground that it presents a significant risk would be a disservice to the safety of users.

Thus, although the committee strongly endorses the FDA's paramount concern for the safety of users of contraceptives, we believe that concern can be most effectively exerted by changing the current standard applied by the FDA for approval of new contraceptives. The proposed change would still impose on contraceptives a safety standard more demanding than that for other drugs and devices (which are not required to show a safety advantage compared with previously approved products).

The committee also recommends that a comprehensive postmarketing surveillance system be established to provide systematic and timely feedback about positive and negative health effects of contraceptive products. Such a system of postmarketing surveillance would ensure that products that are later found to be unsafe are removed from the market or are more strictly controlled through product labeling and health warnings for subpopulations found to be at risk. Systematic and controlled postmarketing surveillance would help to avoid episodes that have occurred with certain intrauterine devices in the United States.

The committee recommends that an international conference of drug regulatory officials be held to increase the priority that such officials give to contraceptive development, to harmonize the regulatory requirements of different countries to the extent possible, to discuss the need for greater postmarketing surveillance of new contraceptives, and to clarify the basis for regulatory decisions in individual countries. Such a conference, in the view of the committee, would make the need for new contraceptives and the opportunities of their development more visible.

The Food and Drug Administration should complete its review of its toxicological requirements for the evaluation of contraceptive products, especially its continued use of the beagle dog. The committee does not recommend any change in toxicological testing requirements that would significantly reduce confidence in the safety of contraceptives or the amount of relevant data that is useful in guiding prescribing decisions. The issue over the beagle dog has turned on whether that model is relevant to the assessment of safety, and whether studies of beagles provide data useful in prescribing steroidal contraceptives for humans. A decision to eliminate that testing requirement would be based on a scientific judgment that the requirement does not add to human safety. The elimination of the requirement on that basis would provide no justification for any change in the principles of products liability otherwise applicable to contraceptive products (see Chapter 8).

A report should be prepared by an independent body three to five years hence to assess FDA requirements with respect to contraceptives. The committee recommends that the FDA continue to evaluate ways to improve the toxicological and clinical trial requirements for contraceptive agents.

Although the committee believes that it is too early to assess the effects of the Drug Price Competition and Patent Term Restoration Act, further study of effective patent life is needed and a report on the effects of the act, with particular reference to contraceptives, should be undertaken in the mid-1990s.

CONCLUSION

Congress and the Food and Drug Administration have made a number of important changes during the past few years, which are likely to influence the course of contraceptive research and development. FDA has revised its regulations governing the early phase of drug research; because most research at this phase does not lead to marketed products or even to extensive additional research, the changes that the FDA has made are intended to reduce delays without reducing the protection of human subjects. The FDA has also reduced the toxicological testing requirements for new contraceptives, which were previously more rigorous than the requirements for most other drugs. The enactment by Congress of the 1984 Drug Price Competition and Patent Term Restoration Act also increases the incentives for new drug development, including development of new contraceptive products.

Although the committee believes that considerable progress has been made in the FDA's regulation of contraceptive products, fundamental questions remain regarding standards of safety and effectiveness applied to contraceptive products.

As argued in Chapter 2, the current array of contraceptives fails to meet the needs of a substantial number of men and women in the United States. Currently available contraceptives present significant risks, have significant failure rates in actual use, make demands on users that many cannot or do not in fact meet, or are inconsistent with the mores, practices, and deep-seated preferences of users or their sexual partners. The results, as discussed in Chapter 2, show that, even in the United States, there is substantial need for better and more varied contraceptive drugs and devices. In particular, some of the contraceptives that are most effective and intrude least in sexual practices—for example, contraceptive steroids, however delivered—are also more risky than less effective methods and, for large groups of women (those over 35 who smoke), carry an added risk or are even contraindicated.

Commissioner Hayes's statement of FDA's safety standard for contraceptives quoted earlier in this chapter does not adequately take into account the number of women who have health conditions for which existing methods are inappropriate or who for personal reasons find the existing methods unacceptable. In saying that contraceptives are used by healthy women, the commissioner does not recognize that a large number of women have contraindications for some available methods of contraception but are not sick as we ordinarily understand that term. For example, nursing mothers, women over the age of 35 who smoke cigarettes, and women with diabetes or hypertension have contraindications for the pill; nevertheless, we would not ordinarily think of these women as unhealthy.

Equally important, in the case of contraceptives, effectiveness must be taken into account in calculations of safety. Methods with fewer side effects are not necessarily safer if they have higher failure rates. The risk of an unwanted or high-risk pregnancy must be weighed in the calculation of the safety of methods. The FDA needs to consider both effectiveness in clinical trials and effectiveness in general use in its approval process for contraceptive drugs. A contraceptive that has a low risk of unwanted pregnancy in actual use is an effective product. When considering the trade-off between benefits and risks, the benefits need to include gains in actual effectiveness when compared with existing methods.

A range of contraceptives is essential to fit the needs of all potential users. Not all clinically effective drugs are effective for all people in actual use. The FDA therefore needs to consider the target population for any proposed drug to evaluate its effectiveness. In other words, a new contraceptive may offer no benefits in effectiveness compared with other methods under ideal conditions, but it may provide increased effectiveness to a particular population ill served by existing methods. This consideration should be given greater weight in the FDA's regulatory evaluations than it has been given in the past.

It is important when evaluating a new contraceptive to compare its overall safety with that of already available methods. Account should be taken not only of new risks presented by the new method, but also of its advantage in not presenting risks known to be presented by the existing methods. For example, the fact that Depo-Provera did not affect coagulation or hypertension (whereas some contraceptive preparations do) was not generally considered in calculations of risks and benefits.

8

Products Liability and Contraceptive Development

This chapter examines recent trends in contraceptive products liability litigation and insurance and evaluates their effect on the pace of development of new contraceptives in the United States. The chapter begins with an overview of the legal environment in which contraceptive products are developed. This discussion is followed by a description of the trends in litigation involving contraceptives, a discussion of current products liability rules, and a summary of selected contraceptive cases. The chapter continues with a description of the products liability insurance environment and, finally, presents the committee's conclusions and recommendations.

THE LEGAL TERRAIN

When a pharmaceutical company or nonprofit organization contemplates development of a new contraceptive, it does not look at products liability rules and cases as isolated phenomena, but at the legal landscape they create. From the perspective of those developing or thinking about developing or marketing a new contraceptive, that landscape can appear intimidating.

First, since all the pharmaceutical firms with the resources to make substantial investments in contraceptive development are national firms that market products on a national basis, they face the prospect of different rules with regard to products liability in each of the 50 states. In practice, there is a good deal of uniformity among the jurisdictions because of the adoption by courts of the *Restatement (Second) of Torts* (American Law Institute and National Conference of Commissioners on Uniform State Laws, 1965), a text containing a general statement and analysis of products liability law, and the *Uniform Commercial Code* (1976), a model set of statutes. Nonetheless, companies operating in a national market continue to face the costly uncertainty that arises because 50 different jurisdictions have the power to make and change products liability rules.

Second, a manufacturer involved in a products liability action will almost always have its case decided by a judge and jury who, although scientifically untrained, must evaluate highly technical and complex scientific issues, often on the basis of only the conflicting testimony of experts retained by the parties. Moreover, judges and juries are much more inclined to be sympathetic to injured plaintiffs, especially mothers and children, than they are to corporate defendants.

Third, if a manufacturer becomes involved in a products liability action, it is not shielded from liability by Food and Drug Administration (FDA) approval of the product.[1] This is so despite the rigorous testing required by the FDA before a new product is marketed, the practice of the FDA to give great weight to safety considerations (see Chapter 7), and the warnings and instructions that the FDA requires be given.

Fourth, both the number of suits and the size of the awards are widely perceived to have increased dramatically in recent years, and future trends are unpredictable. Developers and manufacturers of contraceptives feel that they are substantially more likely to be sued today than in the past and, if they lose, to have to pay (in real terms) more than they would have had to pay in the past. Litigation expenses can be high and are incurred even when claims are meritless. Commercial liability insurance has sometimes proven impossible for some developers and manufacturers to obtain, and very expensive for those who have been able to secure it. The adverse media attention often associated with products liability claims and contraceptive-related injuries may independently discourage manufacturers from research, development, and the marketing of contraceptive products. Apart from the effect of such publicity in stimulating legal claims, the manufacturer may suffer a loss of public confidence in its other unrelated products, even if the manufacturer is not found liable.

SOURCES OF DATA

In an attempt to assess the magnitude and frequency of contraceptive products liability claims in the United States over the past two decades, the committee

---

[1]Recent legislation in New Jersey, Ohio, Oregon, and Texas allows a manufacturer of an FDA-approved product to assert an "FDA defense" in response to a claim for punitive damages—that is, generally the manufacturer cannot be held liable for punitive damages if the product has been manufactured and labeled in accordance with FDA standards unless the manufacturer withheld from or misrepresented to the FDA material and relevant information. Ohio Rev. Code Ann. §2307.80(C) (Page Supp. 1987); 1987 Or. Laws ch. 774 §5, Prod. Liab. Rep. (CCH) para. 93,835; Tex. Civ. Pract. and Rem. Code Ann. §81.001 et seq. (Supp. 1989); 1987 N.J. Laws, ch. 197.

examined a number of data sources. Legal counsel and products liability attorneys were contacted at companies currently marketing contraceptive products in the United States: Ortho Pharmaceutical Corporation; G.D. Searle & Co.; Wyeth Laboratories; Syntex Laboratories, Inc.; Parke-Davis & Co.; Mead Johnson Laboratories; ALZA Corporation, Berlex Laboratories, Inc.; Schmid Laboratories, Inc.; Whitehall Laboratories, Inc.; and GynoPharma, Inc. Representatives of A.H. Robins Company were contacted regarding liability for the Dalkon Shield. Company annual reports and quarterly reports were also reviewed for information on liability claims and recent settlements for contraceptive products. Some drug companies provided fairly detailed information on the number of cases and the magnitude of the awards, while others were reluctant to provide any information.

In order to identify court cases involving products liability of contraceptives, several computer searches were performed using Mead Data Central, Inc.'s LEXIS Service, a computer-assisted legal research service. The LEXIS computer data base consists of decisions of federal courts and most state courts. From the searches it was possible to identify contraceptive products liability cases in which judicial opinions were issued. The number of reported cases, however, is only a subset of the total number of such cases because LEXIS does not identify pending cases or cases decided or settled without a judicial opinion. LEXIS also does not generally produce references to state trial-level cases.

Other traditional legal research sources, such as state and federal topical digests, law review articles, and articles containing case annotations, were also consulted to obtain and confirm data on products liability cases involving contraceptive products. *Pharmaceutical Litigation Reporter, OB/GYN Litigation Reporter,* and *Jury Verdict Information Reports* were also reviewed. A number of independent consumer organizations, lawyers' associations, and victims' network organizations were contacted for additional information on contraceptive liability cases.

Clearly, the committee's search of available data sources did not yield all the products liability actions initiated against contraceptive manufacturers. It also did not identify many of the claims that were settled without initiation of litigation. Because the vast majority of cases are settled out of court for dollar amounts that are unreported and for reasons that are not publicly known, the committee was unable to obtain access to much of the potentially relevant data. In addition, cases decided at the state trial level, whether resulting in judgments for manufacturers or for injured plaintiffs, are usually unpublished; such cases may be published only if and when they are appealed.

Nonetheless, the committee believes that the information assembled on the number of reported cases is broadly indicative of the much larger number of such cases settled without even a court filing, filed but settled, or tried but not appealed. The information gathered is important because it is available to contraceptive manufacturers and may affect their behavior (e.g., changes in labeling) and is also used in settlement decision making to assess the likelihood of success in a particular case.

TRENDS IN LITIGATION INVOLVING CONTRACEPTIVES

Intrauterine devices, oral contraceptives, spermicides, diaphragms, and condoms have all been the subjects of products liability litigation. The IUD litigation has been characterized by extremes: massive liability in the case of one product, the Dalkon Shield, but, with one significant exception of a case still under appeal, limited recovery by plaintiffs in most cases involving other IUDs. The litigation concerning oral contraceptives is characterized by its long-running nature, the adjustments manufacturers have made in response to the lawsuits, and the difficult issues regarding adequate warnings. The one reported case involving a spermicide surprised the legal and scientific communities with a decision that was contrary to currently accepted theories of causation.

Intrauterine Devices

Figure 8.1 shows the number of products liability cases by year that were filed against manufacturers of IUDs and oral contraceptives and reported by the sources surveyed. Prior to 1970 there were no reported products liability cases involving manufacturers of IUDs. The number of reported IUD cases reached its peak during the 1984–1986 period, the same period in which several IUDs were withdrawn from the market and A.H. Robins Company filed for bankruptcy. Prior to 1986, Dalkon Shield cases predominated, representing well over half the

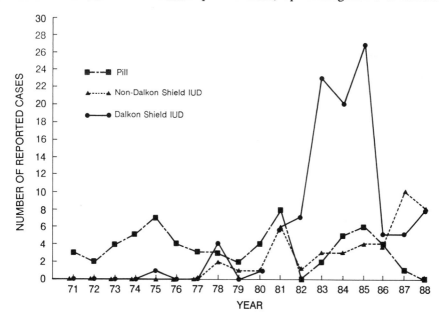

FIGURE 8.1   Yearly reported oral contraceptive and IUD cases.

IUD cases reported by the data sources surveyed. Although the vast majority of cases reported in the sources we surveyed have been settled out of court, a number of cases have gone to trial and punitive damages have been awarded to plaintiffs.

At least six firms have distributed IUDs since the introduction of the first IUD in the United States in 1964. In 1975, A.H. Robins Company stopped selling its controversial Dalkon Shield, and in 1985 Robins filed for bankruptcy after more than 4,000 lawsuits concerning the IUD had been filed against the company. Schmid Laboratories, Inc., withdrew the Saf-T-Coil in 1983. In 1985, Ortho Pharmaceutical Corporation discontinued marketing the Lippes Loop, and in 1986 G.D. Searle & Co. discontinued marketing the Copper-7 and the Tatum-T. With the exception of the Dalkon Shield, all those devices were withdrawn even though the FDA did not raise questions about their safety and very few successful lawsuits had been brought against the manufacturers. Only two firms are currently selling IUDs in the United States. ALZA Corporation has been marketing the Progestasert IUD since 1976, and GynoPharma, Inc., has been marketing the ParaGard IUD (Copper T380A) since 1988. Both IUDs are accompanied by detailed informed consent guidelines.

Oral Contraceptives

Figure 8.1 also shows the number of products liability cases by year that were filed against manufacturers of oral contraceptives and were reported in the sources surveyed. The patterns in reported oral contraceptive cases appear to correspond closely to the patterns in reported IUD cases, with the number of cases peaking during the 1984–1986 period. Assuming the number of reported oral contraceptive cases fairly represents the larger number of such cases filed that are settled or tried but not appealed, they present a picture of manufacturers continuing to market products despite numerous lawsuits.

The litigation against manufacturers of oral contraceptives has persisted over the past 17 years. In sharp contrast to the situation with respect to IUDs, however, oral contraceptives continue to be marketed by seven companies, although over the past two decades manufacturers have complied with an FDA request to remove some standard and high-dose oral contraceptive formulations from the market. Despite the litigation costs, these products continue to be profitable because the market is relatively large and the monthly cost of the pills is high.

Other Contraceptives

Our review of litigation sources identified one case brought against a spermicide manufacturer (1984), one case brought against a diaphragm manufacturer (1988), one case brought against a condom manufacturer (1981), and no cases reported concerning other contraceptive drugs or devices. The plaintiff in the spermicide case was awarded over $5 million in damages. The plaintiff in the diaphragm case received damages of $1.5 million. The condom case, in which the plaintiff sought damages for the "wrongful birth" of twins allegedly caused by the product's failure, was eventually dismissed and the plaintiffs received no damages.

To assist in understanding the impact of such litigation on contraceptive development, we provide a brief introduction to products liability law and substantive summaries of selected cases involving IUDs, oral contraceptives, and other contraceptives.

PRODUCTS LIABILITY RULES

The legal rules regarding products liability that have been applied to the manufacturers of contraceptives are the same ones applied to all other manufacturers, whether of lawnmowers, bicycles, or electric drills. These rules generally have their source in common law, not statutory law; that is, they are rules made for the most part by judges rather than laws enacted by Congress or state legislatures. The objectives of products liability rules are to compensate people injured by unsafe products, to deter the marketing of dangerous or defective products, and to resolve fairly disputes between persons injured by a product and the manufacturer of that product (Smith, 1987).

If, in creating or applying the common law liability rules, courts fail to properly balance the interests of the injured person and the manufacturer, or fail to consider adequately the impact of their rulings on the interests of persons beyond the immediate parties to the litigation, then it is the responsibility of Congress or the state legislatures to correct the balance or account for the wider interests by enacting appropriate laws. Any nonfederal corrective legislation has to be enacted state-by-state, since products liability rules—as with tort law generally—are the subject of the laws of each of the 50 states and the District of Columbia. A federal products liability law, which would preempt state laws, has been proposed (U.S. Congress, 1987), but political agreement on the content of such a measure—and indeed on the wisdom of such a law whatever its form and substance—has been lacking. In the absence of federally mandated uniformity, state legislatures may choose to adopt the Uniform Product Liability Act[2] (U.S. Department of Commerce, 1979; see also Schwartz, 1980), which was drafted to serve as a set of model standards for state products liability law.

A manufacturer of a product may be held liable to an injured user of the product under any one of five legal theories: express warranty, implied warranty, fraudulent misrepresentation, negligence, and strict liability. In most lawsuits,

---

[2]Section 106 of the Uniform Product Liability Act provides that a product seller cannot be found liable on the basis of defective design or failure to warn if the product conformed to an applicable administrative or legislative regulatory standard. This provision does not apply, however, if the claimant can prove by a preponderance of the evidence that a reasonably prudent product seller could and would have taken additional precautions.

plaintiffs endeavor to base their claims on two or more of these theories. The elements of the five theories of liability are summarized below.

Warranty

A warranty claim may be based on an express or an implied warranty theory, or both. An express warranty is a written or oral affirmation of fact or promise made by the seller of the product to the buyer about the condition, efficacy, or safety of the product. An express warranty claim arises when a plaintiff-buyer asserts that the purchased product does not conform to the defendant-seller's representations. Thus, the arguments in many express warranty cases concern (1) whether the seller actually made a statement of fact to the buyer about the product—if the seller merely expressed an opinion, an express warranty claim is not supportable; (2) the meaning or interpretation of any such statement; (3) whether such statement was true or false; and (4) whether the product caused the plaintiff's harm.

An implied warranty is a representation by the seller that is implied in a contract for the sale of the product that the product is "merchantable," that is, "fit for the ordinary purposes for which such goods are used." To recover under the theory of implied warranty, the seller must be a merchant within the statutory definition, and in most states manufacturers have been held to be so (see *Gillespie v. Thomasville Coca-Cola Bottling Co.,* 17 N.C. App. 545, 195 S.E.2d 45, cert. denied, 283 N.C. 393, 196 S.E.2d 275 [1973]). Because all sales are contracts, this theory presents a broad avenue for recovery against sellers of defective goods. Although recovery under a warranty theory against the manufacturer of a defective product in many states has been available in common law for roughly 100 years (Birnbaum, 1980), recovery in most states today is governed by the relevant provisions of the *Uniform Commercial Code,* as adopted by each state.

Fraudulent Misrepresentation

Fraudulent misrepresentation is akin to the warranty theory of liability but has an additional requirement that the plaintiff prove fraud and deceit. In a products liability suit based on fraudulent misrepresentation, the plaintiff must prove the following elements: (1) the defendant made a false representation about the product; (2) the defendant knew the representation was false; (3) the defendant intended to induce the plaintiff to act or refrain from acting on the basis of the representation; (4) the plaintiff justifiably relied on the representation; and (5) the plaintiff was injured thereby [American Law of Products Liability 3d (1987), Vol. 2, §25:1 (Lawyers Co-op. Pub. Co., Rochester, N.Y.)]. Some courts have held that the plaintiff must prove fraud and deceit by "clear and convincing" evidence, rather than by the usual standard of "more likely than not." For this reason, and because of the difficulty of proving that the defendant knowingly misrepresented a fact about the product, products liability lawsuits are not usually based on fraudulent misrepresentation (Id. §25.2).

Negligence

In products liability suits based on negligence theory, plaintiffs must show that: the defendant-manufacturer owed the plaintiff a "duty of care"; the defendant breached this duty of care (acted "unreasonably," was "negligent"); the plaintiff was injured; and the defendant's lack of care was the proximate cause of the injury (Harper et al., 1986). As these rules have been developed in products liability cases, it can be said that today a manufacturer owes a duty of care to avoid an unreasonable risk of harm to the user of the product (Harper et al., 1986). A manufacturer can breach this duty of care in three broad respects: (1) by adopting a design for the product that causes it to be unreasonably dangerous; (2) by making mistakes or omissions in the manufacturing process that result in a properly designed product becoming unreasonably dangerous; (3) or by failing to provide adequate warnings about the product's hazards and instructions concerning its use (Harper et al., 1986). In most jurisdictions the manufacturer must warn only the medical profession, not the patient—the "learned intermediary" rule—and the adequacy of the warning is a matter frequently in contention (Harper et al., 1986).

Strict Liability in Tort

The use of strict liability theory in products liability cases is a relatively recent development, dating from a 1963 decision of the California Supreme Court (*Greenman v. Yuba Power Products, Inc.*, 59 Cal. 2d 57, 377 P.2d 897 [1963]) and the publication in 1965 of section 402A of the *Restatement (Second) of Torts* (American Law Institute and National Conference of Commissioners on Uniform State Laws, 1965). Under a strict liability theory an injured user of a product may recover from the manufacturer without showing that the manufacturer was negligent (breached a duty of care). A strict liability claim may be based on three independent theories: design defect, which includes defective testing; manufacturing defect; and failure to warn. To recover under any of these theories, the plaintiff must show something more than that he or she used the product and was injured by it—but both courts and commentators show a remarkably high degree of uncertainty over the meaning and scope of the doctrine (see Harper et al., 1986; Keeton, 1984; Owen, 1980; Schwartz, 1979).

Section 402A of the *Restatement (Second) of Torts* has had a profound impact on the development of strict liability in the courts. Although intended as a summary statement of common law rules and in no way binding on courts, the *Restatement* has been widely adopted by many jurisdictions. Section 402A imposes liability on a manufacturer if it sells a product "in a defective condition unreasonably dangerous to the user or consumer . . . for physical harm thereby caused to the ultimate user or consumer. . . ." That the manufacturer exercised "all possible care" in designing and manufacturing the product does not absolve it from liability.

Two explanatory notes or comments to section 402A, comment j and comment k, have played important roles in cases involving drugs and medical devices. Comment j states that the manufacturer may prevent the product from being considered "unreasonably dangerous" within the meaning of section 402A by giving appropriate directions or warnings, and (as in negligence cases) a much-contested issue is the adequacy of the warning. Comment k sets forth a special risk-benefit policy applicable to certain drugs that are considered unavoidably unsafe. In particular, provided that the product is properly prepared and marketed and a proper warning is given, a drug that puts the user at a significant risk of harm is not to be considered unreasonably dangerous if the consequences of *not* using the drug also entail substantial risks; thus, the manufacturer should not be held responsible. The rationale of comment k, as explained therein, is that the seller-manufacturer should not be held strictly liable for unfortunate consequences attending a product's use, "merely because he has undertaken to supply the public with an apparently useful and desirable product, attended with a known but apparently reasonable risk." Courts in products liability cases involving drugs frequently employ comment k, and in such cases the only significant issue is usually the adequacy of the warning.

CASE STUDIES

Depending on the facts of the case, one or any combination of these five legal theories can be used by an injured plaintiff as a basis for liability claims against a contraceptive manufacturer. A review of selected contraceptive cases provides insight into the dynamic nature of the legal process. Many of the principles of these cases are reviewed by plaintiffs and defendants to assess the likelihood of success of potential cases. Often, manufacturers appear to adjust product warnings in response to case opinions. Frequently these cases show an alertness by plaintiffs' attorneys to locating and using new scientific studies that may not have achieved general scientific acceptability to contend for more extensive warnings. Cases involving IUDs, oral contraceptives, and other contraceptives are discussed separately, since each product's litigation has exhibited its own distinguishing characteristics.

The Dalkon Shield Intrauterine Device

The development and subsequent withdrawal from the market of the Dalkon Shield merits separate discussion for several reasons: it shows the risks associated with nonregulation of contraceptives because, at the time of its introduction, the Dalkon Shield was not subject to premarketing approval by FDA; it may have influenced the calculations of liability insurers in establishing premiums for contraceptive manufacturers generally and manufacturers of IUDs in particular; and it illustrates the operation of the legal system in addressing the problems raised by a defective product, particularly the compensation of injured persons and the imposition of penalties on the manufacturer of a defective product.

The IUD that was to become known as the Dalkon Shield was invented in 1968 by Irwin S. Lerner, who modified an earlier design by Dr. Hugh J. Davis (*Palmer v. A.H. Robins Co., Inc.*, 684 P.2d 187 [Colo. 1984]). Later that year, Davis began a one-year test of the shield at the family planning clinic he directed. According to Davis, 640 insertions resulted in 5 pregnancies, the equivalent of a 1.1 percent rate during the testing period (Davis, 1970).

In June 1970, A.H. Robins Company purchased all rights to the shield, although two members of its medical department had questioned the validity of Davis's study (*Palmer* at 195). The first reported that the pregnancy rate had climbed to 5.5 percent after 14 months, and the second stated that the period of the study was "not long enough . . . to project with confidence to the population as a whole" (*Palmer* at 195).

A.H. Robins Company began national marketing of the shield in January 1971.[3] In promotional advertising to both the medical profession and the public, Robins made the following claims for the shield: "the modern superior I.U.D."; "lowest pregnancy rate [of] 1.1 %"; and "provides safe, sure, sensible contraception" (*Palmer* at 195–196). In June 1971, a quality-control supervisor at the subsidiary that assembled the shield reported to management that he had performed an experiment that demonstrated that the multifilament tailstring on the shield would wick fluid its entire length, thereby drawing bacteria from the vagina into the uterus of a woman wearing it. No changes were made in the product (*Palmer* at 195–196). From June 1972 to November 1973, Robins received 22 reports of spontaneous septic abortions in shield users, one of which resulted in death, but the firm continued to advise physicians, as late as April 1973, to leave the shield in place in the event of pregnancy (*Palmer* at 196).

In May 1974 the Centers for Disease Control reported to the FDA the results of a survey of physicians regarding IUD-related disease and injury. The survey found that, among patients who conceived with the IUD in place, the incidence of complications was 61.6 percent for the Dalkon Shield, 29.6 percent for the Lippes Loop, and 6.9 percent for the Saf-T-Coil; the majority of these complications were related to pelvic infection (Kahn and Tyler, 1976). One month later, Robins

---

[3]As discussed in Chapter 7, in 1971 the Federal Food, Drug and Cosmetic Act did not require approval by FDA before a medical device could be marketed. FDA could take enforcement action against a device if it could establish that the device was adulterated or misbranded (21 U.S.C. §331(a)-(c), 351, 352 [1970]). In 1976, Congress enacted the Medical Device Amendments, which require premarketing approval for such devices as the Dalkon Shield (Pub. L. No. 94-295, codified at 21 U.S.C. §360-360K).

proposed to the FDA that it voluntarily suspend sales of the Dalkon Shield, and the FDA accepted the proposal. In January 1975, Robins recalled all unsold Dalkon Shields in the United States (A.H. Robins, 1983).

The first verdict in a Dalkon Shield case was returned in February 1975 against Robins for $10,000 in compensatory damages and $75,000 in punitive damages (Couric, 1986). During 1980, Robins incurred over $4 million in litigation expenses and settlements related to the Dalkon Shield (A.H. Robins, 1980). In September 1980, Robins issued a letter to physicians recommending removal of all Dalkon Shields that were still being worn.

After paying $250 million to settle approximately 4,400 suits and after juries in 11 cases had awarded $24.8 million in punitive damages against it, Robins petitioned for protection from creditors under chapter 11 of the Bankruptcy Code on August 21, 1985 (Bureau of National Affairs, 1987). Approximately 320,000 claims were filed by April 30, 1986, the deadline set by the bankruptcy court for filing Dalkon Shield-related claims (Bureau of National Affairs, 1987). In December 1987, Judge Robert Merhige, Jr., of the U.S. District Court for the Eastern District of Virginia, ordered the company to set aside $2.475 billion in its bankruptcy plan of reorganization to compensate claimants injured by the shield (A.H. Robins, 1988).

It is very unlikely that the Dalkon Shield would be approved for distribution and sale today, and it is certain that it would not be approved on the basis of the single premarketing test conducted in 1968. The history of the shield illustrates the operation of the legal rules of products liability, functioning in the absence of premarketing review by FDA, to achieve the objectives of compensation, deterrence, and dispute resolution by causing a defective device to be taken off the market and by providing a mechanism for compensating thousands of women injured by it.

Other Intrauterine Devices

With the exception of one recent case, there has been very limited recovery by plaintiffs from manufacturers of IUDs other than the Dalkon Shield. In the cases summarized below, the manufacturer-defendants prevailed. The first two cases, involving the Copper-7 IUD, show judges and juries struggling with the difficult issue of what caused the plaintiff's injury. The third and fourth cases, involving the Lippes Loop, show plaintiffs seeking recovery from the manufacturer under different theories of liability.

In *Marder v. G.D. Searle & Co.* (630 F. Supp. 1087 [D. Md. 1986]) aff'd sub nom. *Wheelahan v. G.D. Searle and Co.,* 814 F.2d 655 [4th Cir. 1987]), lawsuits by 17 plaintiffs were consolidated into a single case. The plaintiffs alleged that they had suffered three kinds of injuries from wearing the manufacturer-defendant's Copper-7: pelvic inflammatory disease (PID), ectopic pregnancy, and perforation of the uterus. The court held a trial on the general issue of causation; that is, the jury was presented with the question of whether the Copper-7 could have caused injuries of the types alleged, rather than whether it caused particular injuries in identified plaintiffs. When the jury could not reach a verdict, the court declared a mistrial. The court then resolved the issue in favor of the defendant on the ground that the plaintiffs had shown no more than a mere possibility that their injuries were caused by the IUD.

In *Romero v. G.D. Searle & Co.* (15 Prod. Safety & Liab. Rep. [BNA] 669 [D. N.M. 1987]), after the plaintiff had become pregnant she was fitted with a Copper-7 manufactured by the defendant. Her baby was born prematurely while the IUD was in place, and the baby suffered brain damage. The plaintiff alleged that the Copper-7 was the cause of both the premature birth and the brain damage; the jury returned a verdict for the defendant, apparently because the plaintiff failed to carry her burden of proof on the issue of proximate causation.

Beyette v. Ortho Pharmaceutical Corp. (823 F.2d 990 [6th Cir. 1987]) concerned the insertion of a third consecutive Lippes Loop in the plaintiff in 1975. At that time, the package insert stated that the risk of PID with a Lippes Loop was essentially the same as without it. In 1977, in response to an FDA directive, Ortho altered the package insert to warn of an increased risk of PID, and it brought this change to the attention of the plaintiff's physician. The physician, however, did not advise the plaintiff of the change. In 1978, the plaintiff's physician diagnosed her as having severe cervicitis but did not remove the loop. He saw her four more times between July 1978 and January 1979 but did not advise her of the increased risk of PID or remove the loop. In June 1979, the plaintiff was admitted to the hospital with acute PID, and a complete hysterectomy was performed. She sued Ortho on negligence (failure to warn) and express warranty grounds and won a verdict against Ortho at the trial level. The court of appeals reversed. It held that, since Michigan followed the learned intermediary rule, Ortho's duty to warn extended only to the physician, and the company had discharged that duty. Its failure to give an adequate warning prior to the 1975 insertion was not the proximate cause of the plaintiff's injury because of her physician's knowledge and failure to act. Ortho's statement in the package insert about the risks of PID did not constitute a warranty because it was cast in terms of an estimate, and a statement of opinion or estimate is not a basis for a warranty.

In *Collins v. Ortho Pharmaceutical Corp.* (231 Cal. Rptr. 396 [1986]), the plaintiff had been fitted with a Lippes Loop manufactured by the defendant, had suffered pelvic disease, and had undergone a hysterectomy in 1980. The basis for her suit was that the defendant was strictly liable for injuries because the IUD was defectively designed. The California trial court granted summary judgment for the defendant, and the court of appeals affirmed. The court held that, whereas the FDA has approved a prescription drug or device but allows it to be distributed with appropriate warnings of foreseeable risk, such a drug or device falls within comment k of section 402A and thus the manufacturer cannot be held liable under a theory of strict liability for defective design.[4] It should be noted that this decision is not representative of the law in other jurisdictions; in most states, FDA approval does not bar a claim based on design defect, but does serve as evidence in support of a manufacturer's defense.

On January 31, 1986, G.D. Searle & Co., the largest maker of IUDs, announced that it was ceasing to manufacture the Copper-7 and the Tatum-T. The company's stated reasons for its decision were the "high cost of defending unwarranted litigation" and its inability to obtain liability insurance at a reasonable cost (Goldberg, 1986:52,54). At the date of the company's decision, 800 suits were filed against Searle, of which about 500 were settled (Reporter on Human Reproduction and the Law, 1986). As of September 1988, Searle had won 14 of 18 cases that had gone to trial. However, in September 1988 a federal jury in Minnesota awarded a St. Paul woman $8.75 million in damages from Searle on the ground that the company was negligent in testing and marketing its Copper-7 IUD (*Kociemba v. G.D. Searle & Co.,* No. 3-85-1599 [D. Minn. Sept. 13, 1988], 1988 U.S. Dist. LEXIS 10580). This was the first case of punitive damages ($7 million) awarded against a manufacturer of an FDA-approved IUD. It is too early to predict the impact of this case, which is being appealed, on future liability claims against Searle.

Oral Contraceptives

To date, all the oral contraceptive cases that have been reported involve the warning given by the manufacturer concerning side effects of the oral contraceptive. The issues that are litigated fall into three categories: to whom the warning must be given, the adequacy of the warning, and whether an inadequate warning caused the injury.

Nearly all the cases adopt the learned intermediary rule: since oral contraceptives are prescription drugs, the manufacturer has discharged its duty to warn the consumer if it informs the medical profession, including both prescribing and treating physicians, of their potential risks and contraindications (see *MacDonald v. Ortho Pharmaceutical Corp.,* 394 Mass. 131, 475 N.E.2d 65 [O'Connor, J. dissenting], cert. denied 106 S.Ct. 250 [1985]). This information is normally communicated through package inserts and in the *Physicians' Desk Reference,* a physician's guide to prescription and nonprescription pharmaceuticals. Courts in

---

[4]Compare *Ortho Pharmaceutical Corp. v. Heath* (722 P.2d 410 [Colo. 1986]), an oral contraceptive case in which the court held that the trial court properly submitted the case to the jury on a design defect theory of strict liability, despite FDA approval of the drug. The court reversed the case and sent it back to the trial court, however, because the facts entitled the defendant to a comment k instruction on unavoidable risk of harm, and the trial court had not given such an instruction. The case was ultimately settled for $800,000 (Bureau of National Affairs, 1987).

three states, however, have surprised manufacturers by holding that the warning must be given to the user of the contraceptive (*MacDonald v. Ortho Pharmaceutical Corp.*, 394 Mass. 131, 475 N.E.2d 65 [1985]); *Odgers v. Ortho Pharmaceutical Corp.*, 609 F. Supp. 867 [E.D. Mich. 1985]; *Stephens v. G.D. Searle & Co.*, 602 F. Supp. 379 [E.D. Mich. 1985]; *Lukaszewicz v. Ortho Pharmaceutical Corp.*, 510 F. Supp. 961 [E.D. Wisc. 1981]). Courts in Massachusetts and Michigan reasoned that oral contraceptives share many of the characteristics of over-the-counter drugs, and that the users do not rely on the advice of physicians in the same way they do with other prescription drugs. The court in Wisconsin reached the same result by a different route: a federal district court held that, under Wisconsin law, violation of a regulation designed to protect the class of persons of which the plaintiff is a member is negligence per se. The court then held that, since the FDA requires warnings to be furnished to the users of oral contraceptives in the form of package inserts (21 C.F.R. §310.501) and this is a regulation designed to protect the user, the manufacturer had a duty under Wisconsin law to warn the user herself (*Lukaszewicz v. Ortho Pharmaceutical Corp.*, 510 F. Supp. 961 [E.D. Wisc. 1981]).

The scope of the manufacturer's duty has been stated as a duty to warn the medical profession of untoward effects that the manufacturer knows, or has reason to know, are inherent in the use of a drug. This duty requires the manufacturer to keep abreast of developments that could possibly require additional or modified warnings (*McEwen v. Ortho Pharmaceutical Corp.*, 270 Ore. 375, 528 P.2d 522 [1974]). Most courts that have considered the question of the adequacy of a warning have held that compliance with FDA regulations does not, of itself, necessarily constitute an adequate warning; FDA compliance is only to be considered along with all other evidence of whether, in the circumstances, the warning was adequate (*McEwen v. Ortho Pharmaceutical Corp.*; *MacDonald v. Ortho Pharmaceutical Corp.*).

The question of the adequacy of the warning is generally decided by the jury, provided the plaintiff has introduced some substantial evidence of inadequacy. However, many judges have held warnings adequate as a matter of law, thereby preventing juries from considering the issues and resulting in judgments for the defendants.[5] In other cases, there has been sufficient evidence to go to the jury,

---

[5]In the case of *Eiser v. Feldman* (507 N.Y.S.2d 386 [App. Div. 1986]), the plaintiff took Ortho-Novum pills and suffered visual impairment; in *Cobb v. Syntex Laboratories, Inc.* (444 So.2d 203 [La. App. 1984]), the plaintiff took Norinyl 1+50 and suffered a stroke; in *Reeder v. Hammond* (125 Mich. App. 223, 336 N.W.2d 3 [1983]), the plaintiff took Ovral while she was pregnant and gave birth to a retarded child; in *Spinden v. Johnson & Johnson* (177 N.J. Super. 605, 427 A.2d 597 [1981]), the plaintiff took Ortho-Novum and suffered thrombophlebitis and pulmonary embolism; in *Goodson v. Searle Laboratories* (471 F.Supp. 546 [D. Conn. 1978]), the plaintiff took Demulen 21 and suffered a stroke; in *Dunkin v. Syntex Laboratories, Inc.* (443 F.Supp. 121 [W.D. Tenn. 1977]), the plaintiff took Norinyl 1+80 and suffered a stroke; and in *Chambers v. G.D. Searle & Co.* (441 F. Supp. 377 [D. Md. 1975]), aff'd, 567 F.2d 269 [4th Cir. 1977]), the plaintiff took Enovid E and suffered a stroke.

but the jury has found the warning adequate.[6] Nonetheless, a number of cases have found warnings to be inadequate and have held the manufacturer liable:

—One plaintiff took Norinyl and Ortho-Novum pills in 1966 and 1967. In 1968 she suffered hemorrhages in both eyes and became blind in her right eye. In 1966 and 1967 the manufacturer knew or should have known of British studies and U.S. animal studies indicating that injuries such as those suffered by the plaintiff were occurring (*McEwen v. Ortho Pharmaceutical Corp.*).

—A plaintiff began taking Ortho-Novum 2 in 1967 and suffered a stroke in 1971. In 1970 and 1971, the manufacturer knew or should have known of the increased risks presented by oral contraceptives with higher estrogen levels and should have informed physicians of this higher risk (*Brochu v. Ortho Pharmaceutical Corp.*, 642 F.2d 652 [1st Cir. 1981]).

—A plaintiff began taking Norlestrin in December 1975 and died of a stroke 19 days later. The warning was found inadequate because it did not (1) advise of the availability of lower estrogen formula pills that were associated with reduced risk of clotting disorders, (2) advise physicians to inquire about any family history of strokes, (3) advise that a test be administered to detect hypercoagulability before the drug was administered, and (4) advise that women with type A blood are more likely than others to suffer clotting disorders (*May v. Parke Davis and Co.*, 142 Mich. App. 404, 370 N.W.2d 371 [1985]).

—A plaintiff began taking Ortho-Novum pills in 1973 and suffered a stroke in 1976. The manufacturer was held liable because it did not use the word *stroke* in its warnings and in other information directed to the user; the manufacturer did warn of risks of blood clotting (*MacDonald v. Ortho Pharmaceutical Corp.*).

—A plaintiff took Ortho-Novum 1/80 from 1972 until 1976. In 1976 she experienced extremely high blood pressure, hemolytic uremic syndrome, and total kidney failure. Both of her kidneys were removed. The manufacturer did not adequately warn physicians that use of Ortho-Novum 1/80 might cause hemolytic uremic syndrome, malignant hypertension, or acute kidney failure (*Wooderson v. Ortho Pharmaceutical Corp.*, 235 Kan. 387, 681 P.2d 1038, cert. denied, 469 U.S. 965 [1984]). This is one of the very few oral contraceptive cases in which punitive damages were awarded and the award was upheld on appeal.

—A plaintiff died in 1979 from a massive pulmonary embolism after taking Ovral-21. The defendant's warning was found inadequate because it did not stress the risk of thromboembolic disorders resulting from prolonged immobilization or suggest tests for blood coagulation factors, especially in women with type A blood (*Taylor v. Wyeth Laboratories, Inc.*, 139 Mich. App. 389, 362 N.W.2d 293 [1984]).

---

[6]In the case of *Jordan v. Ortho Pharmaceutical Corp.* (696 S.W.2d 228 [Tex. App. 1985]), the plaintiff took Ortho-Novum and developed liver tumors; and in *Lawson v. G.D. Searle & Co.* (64 Ill.2d 543, 356 N.E.2d 779 [1976]), the plaintiff took Enovid and died from multiple pulmonary emboli.

Even if the warning is found to be inadequate, the plaintiff must show that the inadequacy was the proximate cause of her injury. Put another way, if the defendant can show that the plaintiff's injury would have occurred anyway, even if the warning had read the way the plaintiff contends it should have read, then the defendant is not liable. Several cases have absolved manufacturers of liability on this ground.[7]

Other Contraceptives

Only three products liability actions have been reported involving manufacturers of contraceptives other than oral contraceptives or IUDs. The central issue in two cases concerned whether the injury was caused by the product. The third case concerned the determination of recoverable damages.

In *Baroldy v. Ortho Pharmaceutical Corp.* (157 Ariz. 574, 760 P.2d 574 [1988]), a diaphragm manufacturer appealed a $1.5 million award granted to a plaintiff who alleged injury due to toxic shock syndrome (TSS) on a theory of failure to warn. The plaintiff had worn a diaphragm for "extended periods of time" over the course of three days until she developed TSS symptoms. At the time of her use, the manufacturer's patient information booklet stated that it was safe to leave the diaphragm in place for 24 hours and that failure to remove it was not cause for concern. The experts for both parties presented conflicting medical testimony regarding causation, which was resolved in favor of the plaintiff by the jury. The manufacturers argued on appeal that the plaintiff's evidence of causation at the trial was not based on a generally accepted scientific principle.

The appeals court disagreed and decided that there was sufficient evidence presented by both parties in the form of expert testimony and publications for the issue to have been resolved by the jury. The court also upheld the admission, for limited purposes, of subsequent revisions to the manufacturer's patient information booklet; a letter to physicians; and articles, reports, and medical records published subsequent to the plaintiff's injury concerning the possibility of a connection between TSS and extended use of the diaphragm.

Only one products liability case against a spermicide manufacturer has been reported by the sources surveyed, *Wells v. Ortho Pharmaceutical Corp.* (615 F. Supp 262 [N.D. Ga. 1985], aff'd, 788 F.2d 741 [11th Cir. 1986], cert. denied, 93 L.Ed.2d 386 [1986]), and liability was imposed on the manufacturer. In *Wells*, a woman used Ortho-Gynol contraceptive jelly (the active ingredient of which is

---

[7]In *Seley v. G.D. Searle & Co.* (67 Ohio St.2d 192, 423 N.E.2d 831 [1981]), the plaintiff did not inform her prescribing physician that she had suffered from toxemia during her first pregnancy; in *Lawson v. G.D. Searle & Co.* (64 Ill.2d 543, 356 N.E.2d 779 [1976]), the plaintiff was predisposed to blood clots because she was overweight and because of her parity (she had had five children); and in *Vaughn v. G.D. Searle & Co.* (272 Ore. 367, 536 P.2d 1247 [1975], cert. denied, 423 U.S. 1054 [1976]), the plaintiff did not inform her treating physicians of premonitory symptoms of a stroke.

octoxynol-9) before conception and for four months thereafter. Her child was born with no left arm, a partial left shoulder, and a deformed right hand. The mother sued the spermicide's manufacturer, the case was tried before a judge without a jury, and damages in the amount of $5,151,030 were awarded. After presentations of scientific evidence on the issue of causation by each party's expert witnesses, the court found that the defendant's expert witnesses were either biased (several were employed by the manufacturer and others had previously expressed views on the subject), unqualified (had no advanced degrees or specialized training in the relevant disciplines), or did not appear to be credible on cross-examination. None of the defendant's experts had examined the child, and the court seemed to be unfavorably impressed by the omission. Under Georgia law, the plaintiff had only to show that the defendant's product caused her injury by a reasonable degree of medical certainty, and the court found that the plaintiff had met this burden of proof. Having established causation, the court had no difficulty in finding that the defendant had negligently breached its duty to warn users of the possibility of birth defects.

The result in this case, which surprised many members of the scientific community, runs contrary to generally accepted scientific opinion on the issue of causation of birth defects by spermicides. Specifically, two independent advisory review panels commissioned by the FDA had evaluated the safety of octoxynol-9. The FDA's Advisory Review Panel on OTC Contraceptives and Other Vaginal Drug Products in 1978 found octoxynol-9 to be safe (U.S. Department of Health and Human Services, 1980); the FDA's Advisory Committee on Fertility and Maternal Health Drugs in 1983 found no relationship between the spermicide and teratogenic effects and thus found no reason to change the spermicide's labeling (FDA, 1983). In addition, one coauthor of a scientific study relied on by the plaintiffs in proving causation (Jick et al., 1981) reassessed the original study and concluded that the link between a mother's exposure to a spermicide prior to conception and certain birth defects was unsupported by the evidence (Watkins, 1986). Another coauthor questioned the wisdom of publishing the original study in the "present litigious environment" and expressed concern that the article was used as " 'proof' of a causal relationship" without regard to the qualifications and reservations contained in the report (Holmes, 1986:3095; 1987). (See Bracken, 1987, 1985, for other studies pointing to a lack of association between birth defects and spermicides.) It seems clear in this particular lawsuit that the presentation of the evidence by the injured user's expert witnesses was simply more persuasive to the judge than the presentation of evidence by the manufacturer's expert witnesses.

In *J.P.M. and B.M. v. Schmid Laboratories, Inc.* (178 N.J. Super. 122, 428 A.2d 515 [1981]), a husband and wife brought a products liability action against a condom manufacturer on the theories of strict liability, negligence, and warranty. In this case the plaintiffs alleged that the condom was defective and resulted in the birth of healthy twin daughters. The couple sought compensatory damages resulting from the birth of their daughters, including the costs of rearing and educating the children. The appeals court specifically disallowed the specific damage claim for the costs of raising and educating the children. The case was subsequently dismissed and, according to a representative of the manufacturer, no payment was made to the plaintiffs (Kaiser, 1989).

PRODUCTS LIABILITY INSURANCE AND CONTRACEPTIVE DEVELOPMENT

Given the liability and risk inherent in manufacturing and selling all products, contraceptive manufacturers, like manufacturers of any product, seek to protect themselves financially against products liability claims through some form of insurance. Some insurance industry experts consider 1984 and 1985 the worst period in the history of the U.S. insurance industry; in many respects it could be called the worst period for contraceptive products liability insurance in the United States as well. That period saw some contraceptive manufacturers' liability insurance rates more than triple; for certain contraceptive products, liability insurance was totally unavailable; courts approved multimillion dollar awards against a manufacturer of a spermicide and against manufacturers of oral contraceptives and IUDs; at least two pharmaceutical companies withdrew FDA-approved contraceptives from the market; and at least one large pharmaceutical company, which had traditionally been involved in contraceptive development, discontinued research and development of new methods.

Causes of the Insurance Crisis

The reasons for the recent problems of increasing price and lack of availability of comprehensive general liability insurance—which covers products and a range of other liabilities of corporations, municipalities, and nonprofit organizations—are multiple and complex (the reader is referred to the glossary for explanations of some of the technical terms in this section). At least three factors appear to have contributed. First and most fundamental is the underlying upward trend in both the frequency of claims (including products liability and medical malpractice) and the size of awards (Hensler et al., 1987; U.S. Department of Justice, 1986). Second, adjustment to these trends has been exacerbated by interest rates and by the insurance underwriting cycle, in which "soft" insurance markets marked by low premium rates and widespread availability of insurance tend to be followed by "hard" insurance markets in which there are abrupt and dramatic increases in insurance premium rates. The availability of specific types of insurance coverage becomes much more limited in these circumstances. Third, increased unpredictability of future insurance costs results from the unpredictability of tort law in "long tailed" lines of insurance in which liability extends for many years. These factors apply to the liability of developers and manufacturers of contraceptives as well as to medical providers.

Some have contended that the insurance crisis was fabricated by the insurance industry. In 1988 the attorneys general's offices in 19 states filed antitrust lawsuits against major insurance companies, charging that they conspired to limit the availability of commercial general liability insurance (Reske, 1989). Others, pointing to the competitive structure of the insurance industry, have argued that the crisis was caused by the unpredictability of the tort law system and other factors (e.g., Clarke et al., 1988; Priest, 1987; Winter, 1988). It will be years before this issue is resolved; the committee does not take a position in this controversy.

One often-cited factor in the rising cost of liability insurance over the past decade has been the rising size of awards and settlements paid to plaintiffs and litigation expenses (Danzon, 1988). One measure of trends in total costs of liability insurance is incurred losses. Losses incurred on general liability policies rose steadily from about $3 billion in 1975 to $8 billion in 1983 and increased dramatically to $14 billion in 1985 (U.S. Department of Justice, 1986). Harrington (1988) has estimated that the rate of growth of insurance losses incurred between 1984 and 1986 was over 40 percent per year.

The cyclical patterns in insurance markets in the early 1980s have been more extreme than in previous cycles, particularly the swing to a hard market for commercial general liability insurance in 1984–1985. A major distinguishing feature during this period has been increased uncertainty in predicting future liability costs. Two factors are largely responsible: (1) unanticipated trends in tort law, especially the unpredictable size of awards, including awards for punitive damages and (2) judicial interpretations of insurance contracts (albeit in cases other than products liability cases) that have threatened the ability of insurers to contractually limit their exposure. (For environmental liability, see, for example, *Jackson Township Municipal Utilities Authority v. Hartford Accident and Indemnity Co.,* 186 N.J. Super. 156, 451 A.2d 990 [1982]; for directors' and officers' liability, see, for example, *Federal Insurance Co. v. Oak Industries,* Sec. Law Rep. [CCH] para. 92,519 [S.D. Cal. 1986].)

By the nature of the insurance product, the price is set before the costs are known. The ability to form reliable predictions about future costs is therefore critical to the willingness of insurers to write a particular coverage and to the price at which they will write it. The liability system is unpredictable because different courts and juries arrive at different findings with respect to the facts and the appropriate amount of compensatory and punitive damages in similar cases relating to the same product. Unpredictability is particularly severe when liability extends many years after the product is manufactured, introduced into the market, and used. Unpredictability tends to create a risk that cannot be readily diversified through standard insurance mechanisms. Insurers require higher prices for bearing undiversifiable risks.

This climate of unpredictability applies to comprehensive general liability insurance, which includes products liability. In addition, certain types of insurance have been particularly adversely affected. Contraceptive liability tends to be a high-risk category because contraceptives are used by so many women over long periods of time, can create risks that may be latent for years after the product has been discontinued, and can cause severe injuries—birth defects and loss of fertility—that tend to result in very large awards.

Cost and Availability of Liability Insurance for Contraceptives

Contraceptive developers and manufacturers found it difficult to obtain liability insurance coverage during the mid-1980s. This problem was an acute manifestation of the industry-wide price increases and lack of availability of liability insurance. For some pharmaceutical companies and private nonprofit research organizations, the cost of liability insurance coverage more than doubled in a period of only one or two years. For example, liability insurance costs for Family Health International (1985 to 1987) and the Population Council (1982 to 1984) more than doubled during a two-year period (Millaway, 1988; Lynch, 1988). From 1984 to 1988, Stolle Research and Development Corporation gradually decreased its development work on new IUDs, while it continued to observe the IUD liability situation in other companies (Lewis, 1988). According to an FHI representative, the future availability of products liability insurance coverage at FHI is uncertain (Lynch, 1988). For some manufacturers of IUDs, liability insurance was unavailable at any price during the mid-1980s (G.D. Searle & Co., press release, January 31, 1986).

Sharply increased costs of liability and liability insurance can have substantial disruptive effects on the supply of established contraceptives and on the development of new ones. The effects of unanticipated liability costs for products that have already been marketed can be severe. New liability costs associated with products previously marketed cannot be passed on to current consumers of current products. These costs must be paid out of current profits, and thus they erode the flow of funds available to fund research and development.

The effects of dramatic increases in insurance costs for new products can also be severe. Such costs may ultimately be passed on to consumers through higher product prices, but this pass-through is not immediate, particularly when prices for contraceptives are set by public agencies. Nonprofit research organizations involved in contraceptive development are particularly adversely affected; because they do not market products directly to the public, they do not have the power to raise prices, nor do they receive immediate increases in funding to accommodate substantially higher insurance premiums.

In general, if a manufacturer cannot charge a price for a product that is sufficient to cover all costs, including expected liability costs, the product will be withdrawn from the market. In the contraceptive area, G.D. Searle & Co.

withdrew the Copper-7 IUD from the market in 1986 because the "escalating cost of defending unwarranted product litigation makes continuing in the IUD business in the U.S. no longer economically feasible" (G.D. Searle & Co., press release, January 31, 1986). The company stated that the costs of successfully defending four jury trials exceeded $1.5 million, while the total annual sales for the Copper-7 amounted to only $11 million. Almost 500 cases were still pending when Searle withdrew the product from the market, and several hundred more cases have been filed against Searle since the withdrawal of this product.

In the unprecedented hard market situation of the mid-1980s, most insurance companies that previously provided liability insurance for special classes of products such as contraceptives were no longer willing to do so. As the market again softens, it is reasonable to expect that insurance coverage for contraceptives will become more readily available, conditioned on a thorough risk assessment of the product by the insurance company's engineers and scientists, and possibly with limits on the dollar amount of coverage and on other terms of the contract. To some extent, what is reported as a problem of availability of liability insurance for contraceptives may at bottom be a problem of affordability. In theory, there should be some price at which the insurance market would be willing to write coverage for any risk. However, in some cases this price may be unacceptably high to contraceptive developers and manufacturers, given their budgets and the prices that they can charge for their products.

Responses to the Crisis

In response to the liability insurance crisis, a number of adjustments were made in the insurance market. The problems of cost and availability have been resolved in part by a contraction in the market for risk spreading: policy holders are retaining a larger share of the risk through higher deductibles and upper limits of coverage. There is increased use of innovative insurance mechanisms, including self-insurance, captive insurance companies, and risk retention groups, which provide alternatives to traditional insurance and offer advantages to certain types of policy holders. The 1986 amendments to the Product Liability Risk Retention Act have expanded the range of options available and substantially reduced the regulatory costs of using these alternatives.

The contraction in the market for risk spreading seems surprising at first, since the increase in defendants' potential exposure to liability might normally be expected to increase their demand to spread risk through the purchase of insurance. The "solutions" that are being adopted in insurance markets are less than ideal to the extent that they leave the policy holder—or the claimant—bearing more real risk. They do nothing to alleviate the underlying problem of high and unpredictable liability exposure. However, greater risk retention and use of self-insurance may be a preferred second-best solution for some policy holders, given the costs of liability insurance in the face of the unpredictability of future liability costs.

Responses by Insurers

In some situations, insurers have reduced their risk by shifting from the occurrence policy form to the claims-made form. An occurrence liability policy covers claims, no matter when they are made, as long as the injury occurred during the period in which the policy was in effect. A claims-made liability insurance policy covers claims filed within the policy period, for injuries that occurred during the policy period or within the retroactive period defined by the policy. The price of future coverage for claims that may be filed after the policy period but arising from injuries that occurred within the policy period is not guaranteed, but the insurer usually at least guarantees that "tail" coverage will be available. Thus, a claims-made policy shifts the uncertainty of the future liability costs from the insurer to the insured (Danzon, 1985). The claims-made approach was widely adopted for medical malpractice following the difficulties associated with medical malpractice insurance in the mid-1970s, but it has so far not been widely adopted for other commercial classes. Other responses by the insurance companies have been to increase the deductible, increase the premiums, or no longer offer liability coverage for what they consider risky products.

Responses by Policy Holders

The simplest response to high price or lack of availability of liability insurance—short of ceasing to manufacture the product—is self-insurance. The manufacturer sets aside a reserve fund for contingent liabilities; if liability costs turn out to be larger than anticipated, so that the fund is inadequate, any shortfall must be paid out of the manufacturer's other funds or future profits. A manufacturer who self-insures must therefore anticipate liabilities with some degree of accuracy in order to set the price of the product at a level sufficient to finance an adequate reserve fund. To achieve a less extreme form of risk retention, the manufacturer can self-insure for the lower levels of risk and buy coverage only for costs above some very high threshold, provided such "excess" coverage is available.

Representatives of each of the contraceptive manufacturers and developers who spoke to the committee stated that their organizations were unable to obtain, or found it very difficult to obtain, liability insurance and consequently were resorting to some form of self-insurance. Some large pharmaceutical companies are now self-insured for their contraceptive products, for example, G.D. Searle & Co.; Syntex Laboratories, Inc.; Parke-Davis & Co.; and Ortho Pharmaceutical Corporation.

Another form of self-insurance is for a business firm or group of firms to create their own "captive" insurance company. They enjoy regulatory advantages not available to domestic insurers and tax advantages not available to self-insurers. The Planned Parenthood Federation of America and ALZA Corporation (manufacturer of the Progestasert IUD) use captive companies.

A third alternative is the formation of a risk retention group. The federal Product Liability Risk Retention Act of 1981 permits business firms and nonprofit entities that are engaged in similar activities or share similar risks to form a risk retention group solely for the purpose of insuring members of the group. The group may provide product liability and other types of liability insurance. The 1986 amendments extended the scope of the act to cover all commercial liability risks except worker's compensation, and it eased the regulatory requirements on such groups. Essentially, the act preempts state insurance regulation except in the state in which the group is chartered, thereby eliminating the need to be licensed in every state in which a member of the group is located. Several states have enacted special enabling statutes to facilitate the formation of these groups.

Captives, risk retention groups, and other forms of self-insurance share the common feature that more risk is retained by the insured than in traditional commercial insurance. Although there may be some savings to the insured, if these quasi-insurance mechanisms are to be viable in the long run, they must set aside reserves to cover the cost of claims and litigation expenses. Thus, such solutions do not reduce the real risk or cost of tort liability that is faced by contraceptive developers and manufacturers.

Responses by State Legislatures

In some states, legislatures have acted to require increased data reporting by insurance companies and to regulate insurance rates (Danzon, 1988). Such measures do not address the fundamental causes of the problems of cost and availability of liability insurance and could in fact prove to be cumbersome and counterproductive in such a diverse area of insurance as commercial general liability. Even if rate regulation were feasible, evidence in other areas indicates that it tends to exacerbate the problem of lack of availablility of insurance. For example, when malpractice insurance rates were regulated in many states in response to the malpractice insurance crisis of the mid-1970s, at rates below levels considered adequate by insurers, a massive withdrawal of commercial insurers from that market took place (Danzon, 1985). In states in which malpractice rates remain heavily regulated, coverage is still available only through mutual insurance companies and joint underwriting associations, whereas coverage is readily available from commercial carriers in unregulated states. Rate regulation is not a solution that appropriately addresses the underlying problems of unpredictability.

So far, products liability insurance, including liability insurance for contraceptives, has generally not been subject to rate regulation by state insurance departments. Thus, direct regulation of rates cannot explain the lack of availability of liability insurance for some contraceptives in the mid-1980s.

CONCLUSIONS AND RECOMMENDATIONS

From the evidence available to the committee, we conclude that recent products liability litigation and the impact of that litigation on the cost and availability of liability insurance have contributed significantly to the climate of disincentives for the development of contraceptive products. Two aspects of the litigation are especially significant in the context of contraceptives. The first is the unpredictable nature of litigation, which results in part from the absence of stable and uniform national products liability rules and in part from the often erratic character of the litigation system. The second is that, although manufacturers may introduce evidence of compliance with FDA regulations in a contraceptive products liability lawsuit, this evidence is given no special status in most states, such as entitling the manufacturer to a presumption that it acted with due care.

Because of the length of time necessary for development of a new contraceptive product and the costs of development, manufacturers, in considering whether to remain in the contraceptive field, are likely to give the prospects of extensive litigation special importance. Without changes in the products liability rules and procedures, it appears likely that even fewer firms will allocate even fewer resources to contraceptive research and development. The committee makes no recommendations for changes in liability insurance mechanisms. However, concern over the cost and availability of liability insurance is one of the reasons for the recommendations with respect to products liability for contraceptives.

The impact of products liability litigation on contraceptive research and development is a matter of great concern. As noted in Chapter 2, continued contraceptive research and development by U.S. firms is important to the health and welfare of people in the United States and in other, especially less developed, countries. The committee believes that the products liability rules can be changed to remove most of their undue negative consequences for contraceptive development without increasing the health risks of contraceptive users. The committee concludes that an aspect of a contraceptive drug or device that complies with the requirements of federal food and drug law should not be determined to be a defect or a breach of warranty under state law; that the manufacturer of that contraceptive product should not be held negligent for complying with FDA-approved designs or warnings; and therefore that the manufacturer of a specific contraceptive drug or device should not be the source of compensation to someone injured by that aspect of the particular contraceptive drug or device.

Three qualifications are in order. First, the committee has not made a comprehensive study of the products liability system, but has limited its investigation to that system as it affects contraceptive products. It is possible that the committee's proposal could have applicability to all FDA-regulated drugs and medical devices, but our investigation did not go beyond contraceptive drugs and devices. Second, the committee's proposal addresses only the safety, or deterrent, function of products liability law; the important issue of providing adequate compensation to persons injured by defective products is part of the much broader question of the adequacy of existing private and social insurance mechanisms. There are significant gaps and overlaps in the network of insurance programs, and it appears that if different systems of social and medical compensation or insurance existed, the liability rules would be implemented differently. It goes beyond the scope of this report, however, to recommend reforms in these programs or to suggest alternative programs. However, we note that, for purposes of providing compensation, the tort system is much more costly and less equitable than alternate private and social insurance mechanisms. Third, we assume that the FDA will continue to apply high standards in its review of the safety and effectiveness of contraceptives, and that changes made in its requirements for contraceptives (whether those recommended in this report or others) will be fully justified by an appropriate weighing of risks and benefits and are in accordance with statutory mandates.

On the basis of these considerations, the committee therefore recommends that Congress enact a federal products liability statute that gives contraceptive manufacturers credit for approval of contraceptive drugs and devices (and their labeling) by the FDA.

The first part of this recommendation is straightforward: the enactment of a federal products liability statute is intended to deal with the unpredictability and uncertainty caused by requiring manufacturers of nationally marketed contraceptive products to face the possibility of 50 different state liability rules. Of course, a single products liability statute for contraceptives will not completely solve the problem of a diversity of standards in trial courts, both state and federal, across the country. Such a statute, however, would reduce the problem, especially if Congress amended the statute when necessary to assert national uniformity on important points.

The key contribution that a federal statute would make, however, is not so much the reduction of diversity at any given time, as the reduction in unpredictability over time. A system governed by Congress, the Supreme Court, and the 12 federal courts of appeals will produce fewer unpredictable doctrinal trends than one governed by 50 legislatures and state supreme courts.

The second part of the recommendation is intended to address the fact that contraceptive products, as drugs or medical devices, are regulated by a national agency charged with the responsibility of weighing their risks and benefits and having the scientific expertise to execute this charge. Pharmaceuticals and medical devices are unique among products in the United States in the degree to which quality is regulated before they are released into the market. Given that a system of premarketing reviews exists, the necessity for liability as a quality control mechanism is greatly reduced. When the FDA has considered the relevant health and safety data on a contraceptive product, has approved the product, and has required warnings and instructions to accompany the product, it is sound national policy to make this approval available to manufacturers as a defense and not to penalize them for something they could not have known at an earlier point.

In the remainder of this chapter, we describe and explain the sort of statute the committee recommends and discuss the effect such a statute would have on several of the cases discussed earlier in this chapter. Because the statute would interact with postmarketing surveillance efforts, our recommendation would be more compelling if formal postmarketing surveillance studies were generally required.

Possible Elements of a Statute

The extent of the credit that the committee proposes be given for approval of a contraceptive drug or device by the FDA is that, as a general matter, there be no liability for design defect or inadequate warning if the FDA has reviewed and approved the contraceptive product or the warning and has addressed the characteristics of the product that caused the plaintiff's injury. The defense should not be available if the manufacturer withheld relevant information from the FDA in the approval process or if information developed after approval was not reviewed by the FDA for the purpose of determining whether the product or its labeling should be changed. The committee suggests that the proposed statute have five major provisions.

First, if it is established that the injury-causing aspect was in compliance with all applicable requirements of the FDA at the time the contraceptive drug or device was made or sold, then a manufacturer or seller of a contraceptive drug or device would not be liable under any of the relevant legal theories (misrepresentation, negligence, warranty, or strict liability) for any injury related to design; nor would it be liable for a failure to provide an adequate warning or instruction regarding any danger associated with its use; nor would it be liable if the FDA had *not* asserted that the contraceptive drug or device was *not* in compliance.

Second, a determination by the FDA that an aspect of a contraceptive drug or device complies with the requirements of federal law or with FDA requirements would be considered conclusive evidence of such compliance.

Third, the defense would not be available if a claimant is able to establish that the manufacturer should have made design modifications or given different or additional warnings or instructions. Specifically, the defense would not be available if the manufacturer or seller knew or should have known of studies showing an increased risk of harm from the contraceptive drug or device and if consideration of these studies would have led to the conclusion that, without design modification or different warnings, there was an increased likelihood of serious injury occurring to the claimant or persons sharing the claimant's medical characteristics.

Fourth, the defense would continue to be available to contraceptive manufacturers for action after initial FDA review and approval. That is, if a contraceptive manufacturer or seller complies with the FDA directions on the basis of information developed after initial FDA review and approval, then the contraceptive drug or device could not be found defective with respect to any aspects in compliance with the FDA.

Fifth, the defense would not be available if a claimant establishes that the FDA was not informed of dangers regarding the contraceptive drug or device that were known to the manufacturer or seller but not to the FDA and that the claimant's injury is attributable to such dangers.

The FDA Defense

In operation, the FDA defense provided by the proposed statute would work as follows. If a lawsuit is brought alleging injury caused by a contraceptive, the manufacturer of the contraceptive product would have the opportunity to demonstrate that the alleged injury-causing aspect of the product had been reviewed by the FDA and that the agency had not asserted that, by reason of that aspect, the product was adulterated or misbranded or otherwise not fully in compliance with the laws and regulations administered by the FDA. The FDA review may have occurred in connection with an application for premarketing approval (for example, an NDA or PMA), in connection with a §510 submission, or otherwise. If the FDA had not reviewed the alleged injury-causing aspect, then the defense would not be available. This limitation would ensure that state law remains applicable to aspects of contraceptives that have not been subjected to actual FDA review.

If the manufacturer establishes the defense, and the plaintiff does nothing more, the manufacturer would have presented a complete defense, and the lawsuit could be decided before trial by pretrial motion. If, however, the plaintiff seeks to maintain that the manufacturer or seller should have made design modifications or given different warnings, then the burden is on the plaintiff to show by a preponderance of the evidence that: (1) reports or studies showing an increased risk of harm were available to the manufacturer, (2) these reports or studies were scientifically valid or had received acceptability in the relevant scientific community, and (3) a review of these reports or studies should have led a reasonable manufacturer to conclude that design modifications or different or additional warnings or instructions were necessary to avoid the increased likelihood of *serious* injury to the plaintiff or persons sharing the plaintiff's medical characteristics. If the substance of the new reports or studies proffered by the plaintiff were considered by the FDA and the manufacturer had complied with the FDA's directions as a result of that new information, then the manufacturer would be found to have acted reasonably and would prevail.

Effect on Products Liability Cases

What would be the effect of the proposed FDA defense on the specific products liability cases discussed in the chapter? For the most part, the answers must be speculative because of the limited information available: it is difficult to assess the quality of the plaintiff's evidence from an appellate opinion. Moreover, if the FDA defense had been in effect in each case, the plaintiff might have been able to overcome it with other evidence that was available but not adduced at trial. With this qualification in mind, we examine several cases in light of the FDA defense.

In *MacDonald v. Ortho Pharmaceutical Corp.* (394 Mass. 131, 475 N.E.2d 65, cert. denied, 106 S.Ct. 250 [1985]), the court held that the warning regarding possible adverse effects of oral contraceptives must be given to the user and that the adequacy of the warning was a question for the jury, even though it was in compliance with FDA regulations. The plaintiff contended that the warning was inadequate because it did not contain the word *stroke*. This case would almost certainly have been decided in the manufacturer's favor under the FDA defense, because both parties agreed that the warning complied with FDA regulations.

In *Ortho Pharmaceutical Corp. v. Heath* (722 P.2d 410 [Colo. 1986]), the court held that the plaintiff was entitled to a jury instruction regarding liability for design defects even though the drug had been approved by the FDA. This part of the *Heath* case would be changed by the FDA defense; under the evidence presented, there could be no finding of a design defect.

In *McEwen v. Ortho Pharmaceutical Corp.* (528 P.2d 522 [Ore. 1974]), the court held that in 1966 and 1967 when the plaintiff took the defendant's drug, there existed British studies and U.S. animal studies showing that injuries such as the one the plaintiff suffered were caused by oral contraceptives. These studies should have caused the defendant, as a reasonable manufacturer, to change its warning. This case would probably have been decided the same way under the FDA defense; that is, it appears that the plaintiff's evidence would have been sufficient (under the provision that the manufacturer or seller should have made design modifications or given different warnings) to overcome the defense.

In *Wells v. Ortho Pharmaceutical Corp.* (615 F.Supp 262 [N.D. Ga. 1985], aff'd, 788 F.2d 741 [11th Cir. 1986], cert. denied 93 L.Ed.2d 386 [1986]), the court found the defendant liable for failure to warn of possible teratogenic effects from its spermicide despite FDA approval of the warning and despite the fact that two FDA expert panels had reviewed the evidence of causation and had concluded there was no basis for changing the warning. The proposed statute would change the result of this case; compliance with FDA directions would have been a complete defense.

CONCLUSION

The operation of the legal system in this country makes it difficult to make precise forecasts of the extent to which enactment of such a statute would change the perception of the risk of liability, and therefore what contraceptive developers and insurance underwriters will do. As a first step the proposed statute is important, but we recognize that it would take several years before its impact could be evaluated, and modifications may be needed in the future.

We believe that it is important to preserve tort liability for contraceptive products with a few exceptions. The committee did not find that more extreme approaches, such as those proposed by others examining specialized drug development, are called for in the case of contraceptives. For example, an Institute of Medicine (1985) committee studied the problems of vaccine development in the United States; its report proposes a series of options for dealing with problems arising from vaccine-related injury, which includes the option that vaccine-related liability be taken out of the tort law system. We do not believe such action is appropriate with respect to contraceptives. That said, the committee recognizes that, if the proposed FDA defense is enacted and no changes took place in the pace of contraceptive development, other steps might be needed.

The committee believes that the proposed statute constitutes a modest reform and is by no means a radical proposal. It is our belief that a change in the products liability law would change the climate of disincentives for the development of contraceptive products, without compromising the safety of contraceptive use.

9

Contraceptive Development: Obstacles and Opportunities

THE NEED FOR NEW METHODS

Additional contraceptive methods that are safe, effective, and acceptable within the cultural, social, religious, and ethical frameworks of individuals and societies would have a significant positive effect on human well-being. Unlike most other products whose development is regulated by the actions of the marketplace, the development of new contraceptives is influenced by often conflicting and uncoordinated public policies. The impact of these policies, together with other aspects of contraceptive products, such as the complexity of evaluating their risks and benefits and the importance of the social benefits of contraceptive use, has restricted the number of methods currently available and has slowed the development of new methods.

Contraceptive decisions, including the decision not to use contraceptives, must be faced by the vast majority of people of reproductive age. Choices are influenced by a variety of factors, including one's cultural background, socioeconomic status, personal aspirations, health status, and intensely felt individual values. The number and characteristics of available contraceptive methods also influence these decisions and the ability of men and women to regulate fertility in a way that is consistent with their values, economic circumstances, and life-styles. The increasing number of younger men and women in the United States who opt for surgical sterilization as a method of family planning, the high prevalence of abortions, and the very high rate of teenage pregnancy all point to the potential advantages that additional contraceptive methods might yield. More difficult to quantify but equally important reasons to develop new methods are the

147

shortcomings of existing products, including method characteristics related to health risks, effectiveness, and convenience as well as to other user preferences. In short, the health, personal, or economic circumstances of many people mean that they are not well served by existing methods. Noteworthy in this regard are teenagers, women over 35 who smoke, breastfeeding women, and women who have contraindications to the use of most available methods. Often these women are at higher risk during pregnancy and therefore in special need of better contraceptive protection.

Contraceptive use in other societies is also affected by the situation in the United States. Although the methods that would function best in the different circumstances of each developing country vary widely, a broader spectrum of contraceptive methods would have beneficial effects on the fertility, health, and the well-being of people throughout the developing world. Limited contraceptive options have a greater negative impact in developing countries than in the United States because the health risks of pregnancy and childbirth are higher and the social benefits of contraceptive use can be much greater there than in the United States.

The United States has exercised leadership and made significant technological advances in numerous health and development-related areas, but in recent years the field of contraceptive development has not been among them. During the past two decades, scientific and clinical research related to new contraceptive methods has slowed in the United States. Some newer methods or significant improvements in existing methods are now available in Europe, and even in some developing countries, but not in the United States.

Although the distribution of methods, education about their use, and the willingness of couples to use them are all important, the committee concludes that there is a significant need for new methods in the United States, particularly given the mounting public concern over the long-term risks associated with oral contraceptives that have received widespread adverse publicity.

New contraceptive methods cannot be developed in a short time. Development is initiated as advances in understanding of basic reproductive biology are transferred to the clinical arena for testing. The process from that point on is long, arduous, and expensive. Since the introduction almost three decades ago of the pill and the IUD, no fundamentally new contraceptive method has been introduced in the United States. Although the pill and the IUD have been modified to increase their safety and effectiveness, they still are not suitable for use by all couples in all circumstances.

RESEARCH LEADS

New contraceptive methods could become available if greater support for their development existed. Among the promising leads and possibilities are a contraceptive vaccine, long-acting implantable steroids, reversible male and female sterilization, new spermicidal agents with antiviral properties, a once-a-month pill acting as a menses inducer, new ovulation prediction and self-detection methods, and methods interfering with spermatogenesis in the male.

VALUES

The contraceptive choices available to American couples are determined not only by the yield of basic research or the profit margins of pharmaceutical companies, but also by the values people hold, which influence the pace of contraceptive development in this country. Although it is difficult to trace and impossible to measure precisely, our heritage has influenced the attitudes of the nation's scientists, executives, politicians, and the public. The net impact of our values has probably been to slow development efforts and reduce the amount of public support for contraceptive research. There is a pervasive sense among women that not enough attention is paid to the desires and needs of current and potential future users. Some minority group members worry about the potential abuses that promoting contraceptive development may encourage. Whatever the reasons, the nation offers far more support for research to alleviate specific illnesses than to prevent the burdens and trauma of unwanted pregnancy and its medical, psychological, and social consequences.

Most sexually active people in the United States have some experience with contraceptive use and therefore some interest in methods that are safer, more convenient and, overall, more to their liking. To a large extent the problems and prospects of contraceptive development are increasingly discussed by people with strongly held but often poorly informed points of view. If public discussion could be broadened and if potential users felt that their concerns were being addressed in the development process, it is likely that support for development would increase substantially.

ORGANIZATIONS AND RESOURCES

Only one large U.S. pharmaceutical company currently maintains a significant contraceptive research program, and only three European firms support such research. As a consequence, the responsibility for contraceptive development has shifted to the government, nonprofit research organizations, and small firms. This change in organizational structure has contributed to the slowing of the development of new contraceptives. As they have become more active in the contraceptive development process, these organizations have encountered a number of problems, including those related to funding constraints, the limitations of technology, and a lack of experienced personnel.

Nonprofit organizations have begun to play a much more significant role in all aspects of contraceptive development, but these groups face a variety of obstacles that slow their progress significantly. Increased research costs, greater demand for highly skilled professional staff, and the need for better research facilities require long-term financial commitment of a type that nonprofit organizations cannot easily obtain. It is difficult to plan an effective research program aimed at the development of new contraceptives if support for research cannot be guaranteed for more than two or three years at a time. To the extent consistent with the appropriations process, the federal government, which already provides a majority of the funding for these nonprofit groups, should increase funding and adopt arrangements that provide stability for priority research projects.

The committee believes that one of the principal impediments to progress in contraceptive development is the lack of a pool of basic and clinical investigators who are seriously engaged in development efforts. There is a particular need to attract more women and members of minority groups to the field.

Federal funds for training have fluctuated dramatically from year to year and have been severely reduced in recent years. This has led to the perception among young scientists that future work in the field is not secure, a perception that lessens the attractiveness of research in this important area. All but a handful of private foundations do not include basic reproductive research and contraceptive development from their programs. Given the value of new methods and the clear opportunities for research, the committee recommends that efforts be made to increase private-sector support for research on reproductive biology and for contraceptive development. The perception of many is that contraceptive failure and unwanted pregnancy are not significant problems in the United States and abroad—this view needs to be changed. Contraceptives are among the most widely used drugs and devices in the United States and the contraceptive alternatives available to women and men can be substantially improved and expanded.

Since the mid-1970s, federal funding for research in reproductive biology has increased only modestly, and there has been a decrease in the relative funding of applied contraceptive development. Private foundation support for basic research in the reproductive sciences has declined dramatically and steadily since the early 1970s.

Most analysts do not give enough attention to the limitations imposed by the existing base of scientific knowledge on technological innovations. When we understand more about the reproductive process, we may find that fundamentally new approaches of fertility control may arise. The length of time required for development, however, will not necessarily be any shorter. Since basic research represents the underpinning of any future development, support for such research must keep pace with the rising cost of research and development in the United States. The product introduction phase of contraceptive development, which in the past has been substantially neglected, also merits greater attention and increased funding.

REGULATION

The Food and Drug Administration has recently modified the process of approval for contraceptive drugs. FDA regulations for the toxicological and clinical testing of contraceptive steroids have been simplified and the requirements brought into much closer conformity with the guidelines of the World Health Organization and those of other industrialized nations.

The establishment of a worldwide consensus on the appropriateness of regulations governing contraceptives might promote further development. Efforts in this direction could be encouraged by an international conference on the regulation of contraceptive development, from which might come a consensus report for consideration by the FDA and the regulatory bodies of other nations. Although local conditions can and should affect regulatory decisions, the basis for such decisions might be clarified and the quality and benefits of these decisions might be improved through more international interaction.

Present FDA standards assume that contraceptives are used overwhelmingly by healthy people, for whom their use will not interfere with health. In fact, a large number of would-be users have conditions that make them poor candidates for existing contraceptive methods. The adverse consequences of pill use for women with hypertension are one example; the risks and benefits of oral contraceptives for that group are very different from those for other women. Furthermore, the risks of pregnancy, labor, and delivery vary among individuals and populations and are, in most instances, greater than the risks posed by currently available methods of contraception. In addition, some methods have noncontraceptive health benefits; increased attention should be given to such factors as new contraceptive methods are evaluated. However, some contraceptive-related risks are inevitable or unforeseeable. Therefore, greater postmarketing surveillance and long-term epidemiological studies of contraceptives should be undertaken.

The committee supports the rigorous review and approval process provided by the Food and Drug Administration, which adds to the safety of contraceptive practice and public confidence in contraceptive products. The committee believes its recommendations would increase the effective use of contraception in the United States by enabling FDA to approve methods that would allow both users and providers of contraceptives to tailor specific methods more closely to the health conditions and family planning needs of each individual.

LIABILITY

The most frequently cited barrier to the greater availability and faster development of contraceptives is referred to as the liability crisis. The available evidence suggests, however, that the impact of products liability should be evaluated in conjunction with other factors that influence contraceptive development and use. It is important to keep in mind that companies' decisions about what products to market and what research to support are based on a projection of potential profits. Companies stop or do not begin research and development activities, not because of liability per se, but because the potential risk of liability and the costs of protecting against it are not balanced by a sufficiently greater profit potential.

Worries about liability claims relating to contraceptives appear to be particularly important to the major U.S. pharmaceutical companies, as evidenced by their withdrawal from the market of several FDA-approved IUDs. The expense of litigation must be considered within the framework of the rather modest profit margin generated by a contraceptive method, such as the IUD, that does not require repeat purchases. Within this context, it would seem that the private sector has little incentive to develop a product that by modern contraceptive standards would be considered ideal—one that is relatively inexpensive and used only as needed or over a long period without requiring frequent replacement.

The committee concludes that recent products liability litigation and the impact of that litigation on the availability of liability insurance have contributed significantly to a climate of disincentives for the development of new contraceptive products. The committee recommends that certain changes be made in products liability rules to remove some of the negative consequences for contraceptive development without compromising the safety of contraceptive use. Specifically, the committee recommends that Congress enact a products liability statute that establishes uniform standards for products liability lawsuits involving contraceptives and that gives manufacturers of an FDA-reviewed contraceptive product a defense based on FDA's acceptance of that product.

The operation of the legal system in the United States makes it very difficult to forecast precisely the extent to which enactment of the proposed statute would change the perception of liability risk. Although the committee believes that the statute is an important first step, we recognize that it will take several years before its impact can be completely evaluated, and that modifications may be needed.

A FINAL WORD

Our examination of policy issues related to the development of new contraceptives demonstrates that no single factor determines the mix of contraceptive methods available to couples or the speed with which new products are brought to market. While such a conclusion will seem to many readers too obvious to require stating, in our review we found numerous instances of otherwise thoughtful and careful people claiming one or another factor was the sole reason that new contraceptives were not being developed.

Since the first major breakthrough in research on the oral contraceptive in the 1950s, the number of people practicing contraception worldwide has more than tripled to about a half billion in 1988. Because of a rapidly increasing population in the reproductive ages and a tremendous growth in contraceptive practice, concern about side effects and the effectiveness of existing methods and a demand for safer, more effective, convenient, and affordable contraceptives has never been greater. The importance of these issues both in the United States and in other countries is likely to increase even more in the decades to come.

Although not the focus of this report, attention to the factors that would promote contraceptive use among individuals not seeking to become pregnant is also important. New birth control methods—even safer and more effective ones—are of little benefit if they are not accessible, if they are not used, or if they are used improperly. Motivation to control fertility and the ability to use various methods effectively come not only from contraceptive research and development but also from better distribution systems, better education, including education about human sexuality and reproduction, and more open communication about sex and birth control.

Finally, we have not compared contraceptive development to other worthy causes and therefore do not conclude that having a wider variety of contraceptives outweighs all other social goods. However, the committee believes that developing a wider array of safe and effective contraceptives is highly desirable, valuable, and for the social good. In the committee's judgment, increasing funding and other resources devoted to contraceptive development will have an important positive effect, even though the precise scientific and technological breakthroughs cannot be predicted with certainty.

We should move to develop better contraceptives and to work to ensure more appropriate patterns of contraceptive use. New methods can change peoples' motivation to practice contraception. Unless steps are taken now to change public policy related to contraceptive development, contraceptive choice in the next century will not be appreciably different from what it is today.

The continuation of contraceptive research and development by U.S. companies and research institutions is important to the health and well-being of people in the United States and around the world. Encouragement and financial support for American research organizations to initiate, resume, or expand their contraceptive development efforts, as well as reevaluation of and changes in the FDA's mechanisms of assessment of the risks and benefits of contraceptives, and changes in products liability rules will speed the development and introduction of safer, more effective, and more acceptable new contraceptives for the twenty-first century.

References

Adadevoh, Kwaku B.
  1983   Needs for institutional support in developing countries. Pages 213–231 in E.
          Diczfalusy and A. Diczfalusy, eds., *Research on the Regulation of Human
          Fertility*, Volume 1. Copenhagen, Denmark: Scriptor.
A.H. Robins Company
  1980   *1980 Annual Report.* Richmond, Va.: A.H. Robins Company.
  1938   *The Dalkon Shield: Some Questions and Answers.* Richmond, Va.: A.H.
          Robins Company.
  1988   *1988 Annual Report and Form 10-K.* Richmond, Va.: A.H. Robins Company.
Alexander, Nancy J., and Deborah J. Anderson
  1985   Immunologic approaches to fertility regulation. Pages 313–332 in Stephen L.
          Corson, Richard J. Derman, and Louise B. Tyrer, eds., *Fertility Control.*
          Boston, Mass.: Little, Brown and Company.
Alvarez, F., V. Brache, E. Fernandez, B. Guerrero, et al.
  1988   New insights on the mode of action of intrauterine contraceptive devices in
          women. *Fertility and Sterility* 49:768–773.
ALZA Corporation
  1988a   The OROS Technology: A Background Paper. ALZA Corporation, Palo Alto,
          Calif.
  1988b   Transdermal Technology: A Background Paper. ALZA Corporation, Palo
          Alto, Calif.
American Fertility Society
  1986   Ethical considerations of the new reproductive technologies. *Fertility and
          Sterility* 46:Suppl. 1.
American Law Institute and National Conference of Commissioners on Uniform State
          Laws

1965   *Restatement of the Law, Second, Torts.* St. Paul, Minn.: American Law
       Institute Publishers.
Anand, Nitya, and V.P. Kamboj
1983   Role of the pharmaceutical industry of the developing countries in research on
       fertility regulation. Pages 975–986 in E. Diczfalusy and A. Diczfalusy, eds.,
       Research on the Regulation of Human Fertility. Volume 2, Background
       Papers. Copenhagen, Denmark: Scriptor.
Areen, Judith
1985   *Cases and Materials on Family Law,* 2nd ed. Mineola, N.Y.: The Foundation
       Press.
Areen, Judith, Patricia King, Steven Goldberg, and Alexander Morgan Capron
1984   *Law, Science and Medicine.* Mineola, N.Y.: The Foundation Press.
1987   *Law, Science and Medicine: 1987 Supplement.* Mineola, N.Y.: The Foundation
       Press.
Atkinson, Linda E.
1979   Status of funding and costs of reproductive science research and contraceptive
       development. Pages 292–305 in *Contraception: Science, Technology, and
       Application.* Washington, D.C.: National Academy of Sciences.
Atkinson, Linda E., Richard Lincoln, and Jacqueline Darroch Forrest
1985   Worldwide trends in funding for contraceptive research and evaluation. *Family
       Planning Perspectives* 17(5)(September/October):196–207.
1986   The next contraceptive revolution. *Family Planning Perspectives* 18(1)(January/
       February):19–26.
Atkinson, Linda, S. Bruce Schearer, Oscar Harkavy, and Richard Lincoln
1980   Prospects for improved contraception. *Family Planning Perspectives* 12(4)(July/
       August):173–192.
Bardin, Wayne C.
1987   Public sector contraceptive development history, problems and prospects for
       the future. *Technology in Society* 9:289–305.
Baulieu, Etienne-Emile
1985   RU486: An antiprogestin steroid with contraceptive ability in women. Pages
       1–25 in Etienne-Emile Baulieu and Sheldon J. Segal, eds., *The Antiprogestin
       Steroid RU486 and Human Fertility Control.* New York: Plenum Press.
Beck, L.R., and V.Z. Pope
1984   Long-acting injectable Norethistenone contraceptive system: Review of clinical
       studies. *Research Frontiers in Fertility Regulation* 3(2):1–10.
Berelson, Bernard
1969   National family planning programs: Where we stand. Pages 341–387 in S.J.
       Behrman, L. Corsa, and R. Freedman, eds., *Fertility and Family Planning: A
       Worldview.* Ann Arbor: University of Michigan Press.
1978   Demographic Requirements of Fertility Control Technology: 15 Propositions.
       PIACT Paper, No. 1. Program for the Introduction and Adaptation of
       Contraceptive Technology (PIACT), Seattle, Washington.
Berliner, V.R.
1974   U.S. Food and Drug Administration requirements for toxicity testing of
       contraceptive products. *Acta Endocrinologica* 75 (Suppl. 185):40–265.
Billingsley, Andrew
1968   *Black Families in White America.* Englewood, N.J.: Prentice-Hall.

Billy, John O.G.
1979   Accounting for the Availability of Family Planning Services in Counties of the U.S. Paper presented at the annual meeting of the Southern Regional Demographic Group.

Birnbaum, Sheila L.
1980   Unmasking the test for design defect: From negligence [to warranty] to strict liability to negligence. *Vanderbilt Law Review* 33:593–649.

Black, Henry Campbell
1983   *Black's Law Dictionary*, abridged 5th ed. St. Paul, Minn.: West Publishing Co.

Bleich, J. David
1981   *Judaism and Healing*. Hoboken, N.J.: Ktav Publishing House.

Boulier, Bryan
1985   Evaluating Unmet Need for Contraception. Staff Working Paper, No. 679. The World Bank, Washington, D.C.

Bracken, Michael B.
1985   Spermicidal contraceptives and poor reproductive outcomes: The epidemiologic evidence against an association. *American Journal of Obstetrics and Gynecology* 151:552–556.
1987   Vaginal spermicides and congenital disorders: Study reassessed, not retracted. *Journal of the American Medical Association* 257(21):2919.

Brown, Mark G., and Raynold A. Svenson
1988   Measuring R&D productivity. *Research Technology Management* 31(4):11–15.

Bruce, Judith
1987   User's perspectives on contraceptive technology and delivery systems: Highlighting some feminist issues. *Technology in Society* 9(3/4):359–383.

Buckles, R.G.
1979   Contraceptive Product Development in Public-Sector Programs. PIACT Paper No. 3. Program for the Introduction and Adaptation of Contraceptive Technology (PIACT), Seattle, Wash.

Buday, Paul V.
1987   510(k)s and PMAs: Successfully meeting regulatory demands to commercialize medical devices. *Food, Drug and Cosmetic Law Journal* 42:559–566.

Bulatao, Rodolfo A., and Ronald D. Lee, eds.
1983   *Determinants of Fertility in Developing Countries*. Committee on Population and Demography, National Research Council. New York: Academic Press.

Bureau of National Affairs
1987   *Product Safety and Liability Reporter* 15(7)(February 13):139.

Cade, Toni
1970   The Pill: Genocide or liberation. Pages 162–169 in T. Cade, ed., *The Black Woman: An Anthology*. New York: New American Library.

Caldwell, John C., and Pat Caldwell
1988   Is the Asian family planning model suited to Africa? *Studies in Family Planning* 19(1):19–28.

CIBA Pharmaceutical Company
1988   Background Information: The Transdermal Therapeutic System: Revolutionizing Drug Delivery. CIBA Pharmaceutical Company, Summit, N.J.

Clarke, R.N., F.R. Warren-Boulton, D.D. Smith, and M.J. Simon.
  1988   Sources of the crisis in liability insurance: An economic analysis. *Yale Journal of Regulation* 5:367–395.
Contraceptive Research and Development Program (CONRAD)
  1988   Contraceptive Research and Development Program: CONRAD Investigators. Listing of Investigators and Projects, Eastern Virginia Medical School (March).
Cook, Rebecca, S. Bruce Schearer, and Jean Strand
  1982   Contraceptives and Drug Regulation: An International Perspective. PIACT Paper No. 7. Program for the Introduction and Adaptation of Contraceptive Technology (PIACT), Seattle, Washington.
Couric, Emily
  1986   The A.H. Robins saga. *American Bar Association Journal* 72(July 1):56–60.
Crooij, M.J., C.C.A. deNooyer, B.R. Rao, and G.T. Berends, et al.
  1988   Termination of early pregnancy by the 3-Hydroxysteroid Dehydrogenase inhibitor Epostane. *New England Journal of Medicine* 319:813–817.
Danzon, Patricia
  1985   *Medical Malpractice: Theory, Evidence and Public Policy.* Cambridge, Mass.: Harvard University Press.
  1988   Liability Insurance for Contraceptives: Problems in Cost and Availability. Background paper prepared for the Committee on Contraceptive Development, National Research Council.
Davis, Hugh J.
  1970   The shield intrauterine device. *American Journal of Obstetrics and Gynecology* 106(3)(February 1):455–456.
Degler, Carl
  1980   *At Odds.* New York: Oxford University Press.
Department of Census and Statistics (Colombo) and Family Health International
  1987   *Sri Lanka Contraceptive Survey: An Innovative Approach to the Study of Traditional and Modern Contraceptive Practices.* Colombo, Sri Lanka.
Diczfalusy, E.
  1985   Contraceptive futurology or 1984 in 1984. *Contraception* 31(1)(January):1–10.
Diczfalusy, E., ed.
  1977   *Regulation of Human Fertility.* Copenhagen, Denmark: Scriptor.
Diczfalusy, E., and M. Bygdeman
  1987   *Fertility Regulation Today and Tomorrow.* New York: Raven Press.
Dienes, Thomas C.
  1972   *Law, Politics and Birth Control.* Champaign-Urbana: University of Illinois Press.
DiRaddo, J., and W.M. Wardell
  1981   Research activity on systemic contraceptive drugs by the U.S. pharmaceutical industry. *Contraception* 23(4):345–365.
Djerassi, Carl
  1970   Birth control after 1984. *Science* 169:941–951.
  1980   A new look at contraceptive testing. *International Planned Parenthood Federation Bulletin* 14(1)(February):1–2.
  1981   *The Politics of Contraception: Birth Control in the Year 2001,* San Francisco, Calif.: W.H. Freeman and Company.

1983   Future methods of fertility regulation in developing countries: How to make the impossible possible by December 31, 1999. Pages 235–247 in E. Diczfalusy and A. Diczfalusy, eds., *Research on the Regulation of Human Fertility.* Copenhagen, Denmark: Scriptor.

1985   Searching for ideal contraceptives. *Transaction* 23(1)(November/December):41–43.

1987   Contraception in the year 2001. Pages 205–230 in Pieter A. van Keep, Kenneth Ellison Davis, and David de Wied, eds., *Contraception in the Year 2001.* Amsterdam, The Netherlands: Excerpta Medica/Elsevier Science Publishers.

1989   The bitter pill. *Science* 245:356–361.

Donaldson, Peter J.

1981a   Evolution of the Korean family planning system. Pages 222–258 in Robert Repetto et al., eds., *Economic Development, Population Policy, and Demographic Transition in the Republic of Korea.* Cambridge, Mass.: Council on East Asian Studies, Harvard University Press.

1981b   American Catholicism and the international family planning movement. *Population Studies* 42:367–363.

Edelman, D.A.

1983   Development and Testing of Vaginal Contraceptives: Final Report. NIH contract no. NO1-HD-1-2800. Family Health International, Research Triangle Park, N.C.

Eisman, Martin M., and William Wardell

1981   The decline in effective patent life of new drugs. *Research Management* 21(January):18–21.

Ekelman, Karen B., ed.

1988   *New Medical Devices: Invention, Development and Use.* National Academy of Engineering and Institute of Medicine. Washington D.C.: National Academy Press.

Fagley, Richard

1960   *The Population Explosion and Christian Responsibility.* New York: Oxford University Press.

Family Health International

1988   1986–87 Report: Our 16th Anniversary. Family Health International, Research Triangle Park, N.C.

Fathalla, Mahmoud F.

1989   New contraceptive methods and reproductive health. In Sheldon J. Segal, Amy O. Tsui, and Susan M. Rogers, eds., *Demographic and Programmatic Consequences of New Contraceptives: Proceedings of a Conference.* Committee on Population. New York: Plenum Press

Faundes, Anibal

1983   Contraceptive implants: State of the art and prospects for the future. Pages 489–505 in E. Diczfalusy and A. Diczfalusy, eds., *Research on the Regulation of Human Fertility,* Volume 2, Background Papers. Copenhagen, Denmark: Scriptor.

Fawcett, James, ed.

1973   *Psychological Perspectives on Population.* New York: Basic Books.

Feldman, David
  1968   *Marital Relations, Birth Control, and Abortion in Jewish Law.* New York: Schocken Books.
Finkle, Jason L.
  1971   Politics, development strategy and family planning programs in India and Pakistan. *Journal of Comparative Administration* 3:259–295.
Food and Drug Administration (FDA)
  1964   Report of the Public Board of Inquiry on Depo-Provera. FDA Dkt. No. 78N-0124 (October 17):53–54,64.
  1983   Proceedings of the Fertility and Maternal Health Drugs Advisory Committee. Transcript. Food and Drug Administration (December 15).
  1988   *From Test Tube to Patient: New Drug Development in the United States.* FDA Consumer Special Report. HHS Publication No. (FDA) 88-3168(January). Washington, D.C.: Department of Health and Human Services.
Forrest, Jacqueline D.
  1987   Has she or hasn't she? U.S. women's experience with contraception. *Family Planning Perspectives* 19(3):133.
Forrest, Jacqueline D., and Richard R. Fordyce
  1988   U.S. women's contraceptive attitudes and practice: How have they changed in the 1980's? *Family Planning Perspectives* 20(3):112–118.
Forrest, Jacqueline D., and Stanley K. Henshaw
  1983   What U.S. women think and do about contraception. *Family Planning Perspectives* 15(4):157–166.
Frazza, George S.
  1987   Pages 297–298 in Statement Before the Committee on Energy and Commerce, Subcommittee on Commerce, Consumer Protection and Competitiveness.
Free, Michael J., Richard Mahoney, and Gordon W. Perkin
  1983   Transfer of Contraceptive Production Technology to Developing Countries. Pages 189–212 in International Symposium on Research on the Regulation of Human Fertility, Stockholm, Sweden (February).
Freedman, R., and B. Berelson
  1976   The record of family planning programmes. *Studies in Family Planning* 7(January):1.
Galen, Michele
  1986   Birth-control options limited by litigation. *The National Law Journal* 9(6)(October 20):26–28.
General Accounting Office
  1980   *FDC Drug Approval—A Lengthy Process that Delays the Availability of Important New Drugs.* Report to the Subcommittee on Science, Research and Technology, by the Comptroller General of the United States, House Committee on Science and Technology. HRD-80-64 (May 28) Washington, D.C.: General Accounting Office.
Gerson, Kathleen
  1985   *Hard Choices: How Women Decide about Work, Career and Motherhood.* Berkeley: University of California Press.
Gillespie, Duff G., Harry E. Cross, John G. Crowley, and Scott R. Radloff
  1989   Financing the delivery of contraceptives: The challenge of the next twenty years. In Sheldon J. Segal, Amy O. Tsui, and Susan M. Rogers, eds.,

Demographic and Programmatic Consequences of New Contraceptives: Proceedings of a Conference. Committee on Population. New York: Plenum Press.

Glendon, Mary Ann
1987   *Abortion and Divorce in Western Law.* Cambridge, Mass.: Harvard University Press.

Goldberg, Stephanie
1986   Manufacturers take cover. *American Bar Association Journal* 72(July 1):52–55.

Goldenthal, E. I.
1968   Current Views on Safety Evaluation of Drugs. FDA Papers (May):13–18.

Goldscheider, Calvin, and William Mosher
1988   Religious affiliation and contraceptive usage: Changing American patterns, 1955–1982. *Studies in Family Planning* 19(1)(January-February):48–57.

Gordon, Linda
1976   *Woman's Body, Woman's Right: A Social History of Birth Control in America.* New York: Grossman.

Grabowski, Henry G., and John M. Vernon
1983   *The Regulation of Pharmaceuticals: Balancing the Benefits and Risks.* Washington, D.C.: American Enterprise Institute.

Greep, Roy O.
1979   Resources for research. Pages 255–264 in M. Potts and P. Bhwandiwala, eds., *Birth Control: An International Assessment.* Baltimore: University Park Press.

Greep, Roy O., and Marjorie A. Koblinsky
1977   *Frontiers in Reproduction and Fertility Control: A Review of the Reproductive Sciences and Contraceptive Development.* Cambridge, Mass.: MIT Press.

Greep, Roy O., Marjorie A. Koblinsky, and Frederick S. Jaffe
1976   *Reproduction and Human Welfare: A Challenge to Research.* Cambridge, Mass.: MIT Press.

Griliches, Zvi, Ariel Pakes, and Bronwyn H. Hall
1987   The value of patents as indicators of inventive activity. Pages 97–124 in Partha Dasgupta and Paul Stoneman, eds., *Economic Policy and Technological Performance.* Cambridge, Mass.: Cambridge University Press.

Grubb, G., H.B. Peterson, P.M. Layde, and G.L. Rubin
1985   Regret after decision to have tubal sterilization. *Fertility and Sterility* 30:345–350.

Guillemin, R., R. Burgus, and W. Vole
1971   The hypothalamic hypophysiotropic thyrotropin-releasing factor. *Vitamins and Hormones* 29:1–39.

Hagler, Louis, Faye Luscombe, and John Siegfried
1987   A primer on postmarketing surveillance. Committee on Clinical Safety Surveillance of the Medical Section of the Pharmaceutical Manufacturers Association. *Drug Information Journal* 21:69–85. (Philadelphia, Penna.: Drug Information Association.)

Hale, William
1987   Deputy Commissioner for Legal Affairs, North Carolina Department of Insurance. Personal communication with William Campbell (December 9).

Halpern, Sue M.
    1987   RU-486: The unpregnancy pill. *Ms.* (April):56–59.
Haney, Robert
    1974   *Comstockery in America: Patterns of Censorship and Control.* New York: DeCapo Press.
Hansen, Ronald W.
    1974   The pharmaceutical development process: Estimates of current development costs and times and the effects of regulatory changes. In Robert I. Chien, ed., *Issues in Pharmaceutical Economics.* Lexington, Mass.: Lexington Books.
    1980   Pharmaceutical Development Cost by Therapeutic Categories. Graduate School of Management, University of Rochester. Working Paper No. GPB-80-6 (March).
Harkavy, Oscar
    1987   Funding contraceptive development. *Technology in Society* 9(3/4):307–319.
Harper, F., F. James, and O. Gray
    1986   *Torts,* 2d ed. Vol. 3, Vol. 5. Boston: Little, Brown and Company.
Harper, Michael J.K.
    1983   *Birth Control Technologies: Prospects by the Year 2000.* Austin: University of Texas Press.
Harper, Michael J.K., and Barbara Sanford
    1980   Innovative approaches in contraceptive research. Pages 85–102 in Rochelle N. Shain and Carl J. Pauerstein, eds., *Fertility Control: Biologic and Behavioral Aspects.* Hagerstown, Md.: Harper & Row.
Harrington, Scott E.
    1988   Prices and profits in the liability insurance market. In Robert E. Litan and Clifford Winston, eds., *Liability: Perspectives and Policy.* Washington, D.C.: The Brookings Institution.
Harrington, Scott, and Robert E. Litan
    1987   Causes of the liability insurance crisis. *Science* 239:737–741.
Hartmann, Betsy
    1987   *Reproductive Rights and Wrongs: The Global Politics of Population Control and Contraceptive Choice.* New York: Harper & Row.
Haseltine, Florence P., and Arthur A. Campbell
    1986   The Impact of Fellowships Supported by the Andrew W. Mellon Foundation. Internal Report, National Institutes of Health (March 26).
Hatcher, Robert A., Felicia Guest, Felicia Stewart, Gary K. Stewart, James Trussel, and Erica Frank
    1986   *Contraceptive Technology 1986–1987.* New York: Irvington Publishers, Incorporated.
Henry, A., W. Rinehart, and P.T. Piotrow
    1980   Reversing Female Sterilization. *Population Reports* Series C (8).
Henshaw, Stanley K., and Jane Silverman
    1988   The characteristics and prior contraceptive use of U.S. abortion patients. *Family Planning Perspectives* 20(4)(July/August):158–168.
Henshaw, Stanley K., and Susheela Singh
    1986   Sterilization regret among U.S. couples. *Family Planning Perspectives* 18(5):238–240.

Hensler, Deborah R., Mary E. Vaiana, James S. Kakalik, and Mark A. Peterson
1987   *Trends in Tort Litigation: The Story Behind the Statistics.* R-3583-1CJ. Santa Monica, Calif.: The RAND Corp.

Herz, Barbara, and Anthony R. Measham
1987   The Safe Motherhood Initiative: Proposals for Action. Discussion Paper, no. 9. The World Bank, Washington, D.C.

Himes, Norman
1936   *Medical History of Contraception.* New York: Schocken Books.

Hobcraft, John
1987   Does Family Planning Save Children's Lives? Paper prepared for the Conference on Better Health for Women and Children Through Family Planning, Nairobi, Kenya, October 5-6.

Holmes, Lewis B.
1986   Vaginal spermicides and congenital disorders: The validity of a study. *Journal of the American Medical Association* 256(22)(December 12):3096.
1987   Vaginal spermicides and congenital disorders: study reassessed, not retracted. *Journal of the American Medical Association* 257(21)(June 5):2919.

Hulka, Barbara S., and Nicholas Wright
1981   *Contraceptive Evaluation: An Evaluation and Assessment of the State of the Science.* National Institute of Child Health and Human Development. Washington, D.C.: U.S. Department of Health and Human Services.

Institute for International Studies in Natural Family Planning (IISNFP)
1988   Technical Progress Report: October 1, 1987–March 31, 1988. Georgetown University, Washington D.C.

Institute of Medicine
1985   *Vaccine Supply and Innovation.* Washington, D.C.: National Academy Press.

International Planned Parenthood Federation (IPPF)
1988   Femshield—A new barrier contraceptive for women. *Medical Bulletin* 22(3)(June):4.

Issacs, Stephen L.
1981   *Population Law and Policy.* New York: Human Sciences Press.

Isaacs, Stephen L., and Renee Holt
1987a   Contraceptive technology and the law. *Technology in Society* 9(3/4):339-358.
1987b   Drug regulation, product liability, and the contraceptive crunch: Choices are dwindling. *Journal of Legal Medicine* 8:533-553.

Janowitz, Barbara, J.E. Higgins, D.L. Clopton, M.S. Nakumura, and M.L. Brown
1982   Access to post-partum sterilization in southeast Brazil. *Medical Care* 20(5):526.

Janowitz, Barbara, Thomas T. Kane, Jose Maria Arruda, Deborah Covington, and Leo Morris
1986   Side effects and discontinuation of oral contraceptive use in southern Brazil. *Journal of Biosocial Science* 18:261-271.

Jick, Hershel, Alexander M. Walker, Kenneth J. Rothman, Judith R. Hunter, Lewis B. Holmes, Richard N. Watkins, Diane C. D'Ewart, Anne Danford, and Sue Madsen
1981   Vaginal spermicides and congenital disorders. *Journal of the American Medical Association* 245(13)(April 3):1329.

Joffe, Carole
    1986   *The Regulation of Sexuality: Experiences of Family Planning Workers.*
            Philadelphia, Penna.: Temple University Press.
Johansson, Elof D.B.
    1987   The future of contraceptive technology. *Technology in Society* 9:283–288.
John D. and Catherine T. MacArthur Foundation
    1987   *Annual Report.* Chicago, Ill.: MacArthur Foundation.
Kahn, Henry S., and Carl W. Tyler, Jr.
    1976   An association between the Dalkon Shield and complicated pregnancies among
            women hospitalized for intrauterine contraceptive device-related disorders.
            American Journal of Obstetrics and Gynecology 125(1)(May):83–86.
Kaiser, Robert
    1989   Vice President and General Counsel, London International U.S. Holdings, Inc.
            Personal communication (May 26).
Kaitin, Kenneth I., and A. Gene Trimble
    1987   Implementation of the Drug Price Competition and Patent Term Restoration
            Act of 1984:   A progress report. *Journal of Clinical Research and Drug
            Development* 1:263–275.
Kaitin, Kenneth I., Barbara W. Richard, and Louis Lasagna
    1987   Trends in drug development: The 1985–86 new drug approvals. *Journal of
            Clinical Pharmacology* 27(8):542–548.
Keeton, W. Page, ed.
    1984   *Prosser and Keaton on the Law of Torts.* Fifth edition. St. Paul, Minn.: West
            Publishing Co.
Kellner, Menachem Marc, ed.
    1978   *Contemporary Jewish Ethics.* New York: Sanhedrin Press.
Kennedy, David
    1970   *Birth Control in America: The Career of Margaret Sanger.* New Haven,
            Conn.: Yale University Press.
Kertzer, Rabbi Morris N.
    1978   *What is a Jew?* Fourth ed. New York: Collier Books.
Kessler, Alexander
    1983   Manpower and facilities for research in family planning. Pages 179–188 in E.
            Diczfalusy and A. Diczfalusy, eds., *Research on the Regulation of Human
            Fertility,* Volume 1. Copenhagen, Denmark: Scriptor.
Kimble, William, and Robert O. Lesher
    1979   *Products Liability.* St. Paul, Minn.: West Publishing Company.
Kleinman, Ronald L., ed.
    1988   *1988 Directory of Hormonal Contraceptives.* London, England: International
            Planned Parenthood Federation (IPPF) International Office.
Klitsch, Michael
    1988   The return of the IUD. *Family Planning Perspectives* 20(1)(January/
            February):19–40.
Knodel, John, Tony Bennett, and Suthon Pamyadilok
    1983   *Providing Pills Free: Does It Make a Difference? Thailand's Experience With
            a Free Pill Policy.* Research Reports, no. 83-46. Ann Arbor, Mich.: Population
            Studies Center, University of Michigan.

Laing, John E.
1978   Estimating the effects of contraceptive use on fertility: Techniques and findings from the 1974 Philippine National Acceptor Survey. *Studies in Family Planning* 9(6):150–162.

Lamanna, Mary Ann
1984   Social sciences and ethical issues: The policy implications of poll data on abortion. In S. Callahan and D. Callahan, eds., *Abortion: Understanding Differences*. New York: Plenum Press.

Lane, M.E., R. Arceo, and A.J. Sobrero
1976   Successful use of the diaphragm and jelly by a young population: Report. *Family Planning Perspectives* 6(2):61–86.

Lapham, Robert J., and W. Parker Mauldin
1987   The effects of family planning on fertility: Research findings. Pages 647–680 in Robert J. Lapham and George B. Simmons, eds., *Organizing for Effective Family Planning Programs*. Washington, D.C.: National Academy Press.

Lapham, Robert J., and George B. Simmons, eds.
1987   *Organization for Effective Family Planning Programs*. Working Group on Family Planning Effectiveness. Washington, D.C.: National Academy Press.

Lasagna, Louis, and Lars Werko
1986   International differences in drug regulation philosophy. *International Journal of Technology Assessment in Health Care* 2:615–618.

Lee, Nancy C., Herbert B. Peterson, and Susan Y. Chu
1989   Health effects of contraception. In A. Parnell, ed., *Contraception and Reproduction: Health Consequences for Women and Children in the Developing World. Background Papers*. Washington, D.C.: National Academy Press.

Leiras Pharmaceuticals
1986   *Norplant® Contraceptive Implants*. Turku, Finland: Leiras Medica.

Lettenmaier, Cheryl, Laurie Liskin, Cathleen A. Church, and John A. Harris
1988   Mother's lives matter: Maternal health in the community. *Population Reports* Series L (September) (7).

Levin, Richard C.
1986   A new look at the patent system. *Area Papers and Proceedings* 76(2):199–202.
1988   Appropriability, R&D spending, and technological performance. *American Economic Review* 78(2)(May):424–428.

Lewis, Daniel
1988   Executive Vice President, New Product Development, Stolle R&D Corp. Personal communication (March 4).

Lincoln, Richard, and Lisa Kaeser
1987   Whatever happened to the contraceptive revolution? *International Family Planning Perspectives* 13(4)(December):141–145.

Liskin, Laurie, and Richard Blackburn
1987   Hormonal contraception: New long-acting methods. *Population Reports* (March–April):K-3:K-57-K-87.

Liskin, Laurie, and Ward Rinehart
1985   Minilaparotomy and laparoscopy: Safe, effective, and widely used. *Population Reports* (May):C-9:C-125-C-167.

Littlewood, Thomas B.
   1977   *The Politics of Birth Control.* Notre Dame, Ind.: University of Notre Dame Press.
Luker, Kristin
   1984a   Abortion and the meaning of life. In S. Callahan and D. Callahan, eds., *Abortion: Understanding Differences.* New York: Plenum Press.
   1984b   *Abortion and the Politics of Motherhood.* Berkeley: University of California Press.
Lumbroso, Alex
   1981   The introduction of new drugs. Pages 61–77 in Richard Blum, Andrew Herxheimer, Catherine Stenzl, and Jasper Woodcock, eds., *Pharmaceuticals and Health Policy.* New York: Holmes and Meier Publishers, Inc.
Luukkainen, T., J. Toivonen, and P. Lahteenmaki
   1987   Medicated intrauterine devices. Pages 153–163 in E. Diczfalusy and M. Bygdeman, eds., *Fertility Regulation Today and Tomorrow.* New York: Raven Press.
Lynch, Clay
   1988   Senior Accountant, Family Health International. Personal communication (May 27).
Maine, D., and A. Rosenfield
   1982   Maternal and child health benefits of family planning. Pages 1–12 in J.J. Sciarra, ed., *Gynecology and Obstetrics.* Hagerstown, Md.: Harper & Row.
Malyk, B., and J.W. Kompare
   1983   Contraceptive Efficacy Study of 2% Nonoxynol-9 gel with Diaphragm. June 17. Ortho Pharmaceutical, Raritan, N.J.
Mansfield, Edwin
   1986   Patents and innovation: An empirical study. *Management Science* 32:(2)173–181.
Mastroianni, L., Jr., and C.H. Rosseau
   1965   Influence of the intrauterine coil on ovum transport and sperm distribution in the monkey. *American Journal of Obstetrics and Gynecology* 93:416–420.
Mattison, Nancy, A. Gene Trimble, and Louis Lasagna
   1988   New drug development in the United States, 1963 through 1984. *Clinical Pharmacology and Therapeutics* 43 (March):290–301.
Mauldin, W. Parker, and Sheldon J. Segal
   1986   *Prevalence of Contraceptive Use in Developing Countries.* New York: Rockefeller Foundation.
McGarity, Thomas O.
   1985   The role of regulatory analysis in regulatory decision making. Pages 107–364 in *Administrative Conference of the United States: Recommendations and Reports.* U.S. Government Printing Office Supt. Doc. no. 1986-153-115:50200. Washington, D.C.: Administrative Conference of the United States.
Millaway, Elsie
   1988   Population Council Accounting Office. Personal Communication (June 1).
Mohr, James C.
   1978   *Abortion in America: The Origins & Evolutions of National Policy 1800–1900.* New York: Oxford University Press.

Morrow, Margaret M., Michael J. Free, and Richard T. Mahoney
  1988   The changing climate for the private sector. In *Advancement of Indian Technologies for Reproductive and Other Health Applications*. Report prepared for U.S. AID by the Program for the Introduction of Contraceptive Technology (PIACT).

Munsey, R., and F. Samuel, Jr.
  1984   Medical Device Regulation in Transition. Pages 350–379 in Gary L. Yingling, ed., *Seventy-Fifth Anniversary Commemorative Volume of Food and Drug Law*. Washington, D.C.: Food and Drug Law Institute.

Murphy, Francis
  1981   Catholic perspectives on population issues II. *Population Bulletin* 35(6).

Mutambirwa, Jane
  1988   Users' Perspectives in Contraceptive Development. Background paper prepared for the Committee on Contraceptive Development, National Research Council and Institute of Medicine.

National Academy of Engineering
  1983   *Competitive Status of U.S. Pharmaceutical Industry*. Pharmaceutical Panel, Committee on Technology and International Economic and Trade Issues. Washington, D.C.: National Academy Press.

National Academy of Sciences
  1987   *Science and Technology Centers: Principles and Guidelines*. Panel on Science and Technology Centers. Washington, D.C.: National Academy Press.

National Research Council
  1986   *Population Growth and Economic Development: Policy Questions*. Washington, D.C.: National Academy Press.
  1989   *Contraception and Reproduction: Health Consequences for Women and Children in the Developing World*. Washington, D.C.: National Academy Press.

National Research Council, Commission on Life Sciences
  1979   *Contraception: Science, Technology, and Application*. Washington D.C.: National Academy of Sciences.
  1983   *Risk Assessment in the Federal Government: Managing the Process*. Committee on Institutional Means for Assessment of Risks to Public Health. Washington, D.C.: National Academy Press.

National Science Foundation
  1984   *Assessment of the Industry/University Cooperative Research Projects Program (IUCR)*. (November) Volume. 1., Washington, D.C.: National Science Foundation.

National Women's Health Network
  1988   The Network News. (January/February).

Nieman, L.K., T.M. Choate, G.P. Chrousos, D.L. Healy, M. Morin, D. Renquist, G.R. Merriam, I.M. Spitz, C.W. Bardin, E. Baulieu, and D.L. Loriaux.
  1987   The progesterone antagonist RU486: A potential new contraceptive agent. *New England Journal of Medicine* 316:187–191.

Noonan, John
  1965   *Contraception: A History of Its Treatment by the Catholic Theologians and Canonists*. Cambridge, Mass.: Belknap Press of Harvard University Press.

Office of Technology Assessment
    1981   *World Population and Fertility Planning Technologies: The Next 20 Years.*
            Washington, D.C.: Office of Technology Assessment.
Ory, Howard W., Jacqueline D. Forrest, and Richard Lincoln
    1983   *Making Choices: Evaluating the Health Risks and Benefits of Birth Control
            Methods.* New York: The Alan Guttmacher Institute.
Owen, David G.
    1980   Rethinking the policies of strict products liability. *Vanderbilt Law Review*
            33:680–715.
Pasquale, Samuel A.
    1980   Evaluation of new contraceptives: A study design. Pages 2–12 in Gerald I.
            Zatuchni, Miriam H. Labbok, and John J. Sciarra, eds., *Research Frontiers in
            Fertility Regulation.* Hagerstown, Md.: Harper & Row.
Pauerstein, Carl J.
    1980   Some considerations concerning the design and interpretation of clinical trials.
            Pages 37–48 in Gerald I. Zatuchni, Miriam H. Labbok, and John J.Sciarra, eds.,
            Research Frontiers in Fertility Regulation. Hagerstown, Md.: Harper & Row.
Petchesky, Rosalind P.
    1984   *Abortion and Woman's Choice: The State, Sexuality and Reproductive Freedom.*
            New York: Longman.
Pettiti, Diana B.
    1985   Statistical aspects of the evaluation of the safety and effectiveness of fertility
            control methods. Pages 313–332 in Stephen L. Corson, Richard J. Derman,
            and Louise B. Tyrer, eds., *Fertility Control.* Boston, Mass.: Little, Brown and
            Co.
Pharmaceutical Manufacturers Association
    1987   *1987 Annual Report.* Washington, D.C.: Pharmaceutical Manufacturers
            Association.
Phillips, James F., Mian Bazle Hossain, A.A. Zahidul Hugue, and Jalaluddin Akbar
    1989   A case study of contraceptive introduction: Domiciliary depot-medroxy
            progesterone acetate services in rural Bangladesh. In Sheldon J. Segal, Amy O.
            Tsui, and Susan M. Rogers, eds., *Demographic and Programmatic
            Consequences of New Contraceptives: Proceedings of a Conference.* Committee
            on Population. New York: Plenum Press.
Pines, Wayne L.
    1981   *A Primer on New Drug Development.* HEW Publication No. (FDA) 81-3021.
            Washington, D.C.: U.S. Food and Drug Administration.
Population Council
    1986   *Norplant® Worldwide* No. 5 (August). New York: The Population Council.
    1988   *1987 Annual Report.* New York: The Population Council.
Population Crisis Committee
    1985   Issues in contraceptive development. *Population Briefing Sheets* No. 15 (May).
Potts, Malcolm
    1988   Birth control methods in the United States. *Family Planning Perspectives*
            20(6)(November/December):288–297.
Potts, Malcolm, and Richard Lincoln
    1988   Is Contraception at the End of the Line? Background paper prepared for the
            Committee on Contraceptive Development, National Research Council and
            Institute of Medicine.

Priest, George L.
1987 The current insurance crisis and modern tort law. *Yale Law Journal* 96(June):1521–1590.

Program for Applied Research on Fertility Regulation (PARFR)
1985 Phase II clinical study of implanted Norithindrone pellets for long-term contraception in women. *Advances in Contraception* 1(4):295–304.
1987 *Program for Applied Research on Fertility Regulation: Final Report July 1, 1986–June 30, 1987.* Chicago: Northwestern University.

Program for the Introduction and Adaptation of Contraceptive Technology (PIACT)/ PATH
1988 FDA confirms new requirements for steroid testing. *Outlook* 6(1):10.

Ratzinger, J., and A. Bovone
1987 *Congregation for the Doctrine of the Faith: Instruction on the Dignity of Procreation.* Rome, Italy: Vatican Polyglot Press.

Reed, James
1978 *The Birth Control Movement and American Society—From Private Vice to Public Virtue.* Princeton, N.J.: Princeton University Press.

Reporter on Human Reproduction and the Law
1986 (January-February):13.

Reske, Henry J.
1989 Was there a liability crisis? *American Bar Association Journal* 75(January): 46–50.

Richard, Barbara W., and Louis Lasagna
1987 Drug regulation in the United States and the United Kingdom: the Depo-Provera story. *Annals of Internal Medicine* (June) 106:886–891.

Rivera, R., C. Flores, S. Aldaba, and A. Hernandez
1984 Norethisterone microspheres 6-month system: Clinical results. Pages 418–424 in G.I. Zatuchni, A. Goldsmith, J.D. Shelton, and J.J. Sciarra, eds., *Long-acting Contraceptive Delivery Systems.* Philadelphia: Harper & Row.

Rosenfield, Allan G., and Charoon Limcharoen
1972 Auxiliary midwife prescription of oral contraceptives. *American Journal of Obstetrics and Gynecology* 114(7):942–949.

Rosner, Fred
1986 *Modern Medicine and Jewish Ethics.* New York: Yeshiva University Press.

Ross, John A.
1983 Birth control methods and their effects on fertility. Pages 54–88 in Rodolfo A. Bulatao and Ronald D. Lee, eds., *Determinants of Fertility in Developing Countries, Volume 2, Fertility Regulation and Institutional Influence.* New York: Academic Press.

Rossi, Alice S., and Bhavani Sitaraman
1988 Abortion in context: Historical trends and future changes. *Family Planning Perspectives* 20(6)(November/December):273–281.

Rovner, Sandy
1987 FDA panel urges approval of U.S. sales of cervical cap. *The Washington Post* (February 25).

Rowe, Patrick J.
1983 A review of drug registration requirements for fertility regulating methods. Pages 324–335 in E. Diczfalusy and A. Diczfalusy, eds., *Research on the Regulation of Human Fertility,* Volume 1. Copenhagen, Denmark: Scriptor.

Ryder, N.B.
    1973   Contraceptive failure in the United States. *Family Planning Perspectives* 5(3):133–142.
Schally, A.V., A. Arimura, Y. Baba, R.M. Nair, H. Matsuo, T.W. Redding, and L. Debeljuk
    1971   Isolation and properties of the FSH and LH-releasing hormone. *Biochemical and Biophysics Research Communications* 16:392–399.
Schirm, A.L., J. Trussell, J. Menken, and W.R. Grady
    1982   Contraceptive failure in the United States: The impact of social, economic, and demographic factors. *Family Planning Perspectives* 14(2):68–73.
Schwartz, Gary T.
    1979   Foreword: Understanding products liability. *California Law Review* 67:435–496.
Schwartz, Victor E.
    1980   The Uniform Product Liability Act—A brief overview. *Vanderbilt Law Review* 33:579–592.
Scrimshaw, Susan, P. Engle, L. Ross, and K. Haynes
    1987   Factors affecting breastfeeding among Mexican women in Los Angeles. *American Journal of Public Health* 77(4):467–470.
Scrip
    1987   U.S. market projections to 1991. *Scrip* 1180:18.
Seaman, Barbara
    1980a   *Female and Free: The Sex Life of the Contemporary Woman.* New York: Random House (Fawcett Books).
    1980b   *The Doctor's Case Against the Pill.* Garden City, N.Y.: Doubleday.
Segal, Sheldon J.
    1987   The development of modern contraceptive technology. *Technology in Society* 9:277–282.
    1989   Contraceptive innovations: Needs and opportunities. In Sheldon J. Segal, Amy O. Tsui, and Susan M. Rogers, eds., *Demographic and Programmatic Consequences of New Contraceptives: Proceedings of a Conference.* Committee on Population. New York: Plenum Press.
Segal, Sheldon J., Amy O. Tsui, and Susan M. Rogers, eds.
    1989   *Demographic and Programmatic Consequences of New Contraceptives: Proceedings of a Conference.* Committee on Population. New York: Plenum Press.
Shain, Rochelle N., Warren P. Miller, and Alan E. C. Holden
    1984   The decision to terminate childbearing: Differences in preoperative ambivalence between tubal ligation women and vasectomy wives. *Social Biology* 31(1–2): 40–58.
Shaw, Jane E., and John Urquhart
    1981   Transdermal drug administration—A nuisance becomes an opportunity. *British Medical Journal* 283 (October 3):875–876.
    1988   Programmed, systemic drug delivery by the transdermal route. Palo Alto, Calif.: ALZA Corporation.
Sherris, Jacqueline D.
    1984   New developments in vaginal contraception. *Population Reports* (January-February) H-7:H-157-H-190.

Sivin, I., and H.J. Tatum
  1981   Four years of experience with the TW-380A intrauterine contraceptive device. *Fertility and Sterility* 36:159–163.
Smith, Steven D.
  1987   The critics and the "crisis": A reassessment of current conceptions of tort law. *Cornell Law Review* 72:765–798.
Stephen, Elizabeth H., and Apichat Chamratrithirong
  1988   Contraceptive side effects among current users in Thailand. *International Family Planning Perspectives* 14(1):9–14.
Strandberg, Kjell
  1985   Experiences from the WHO Collaboratoring Centre for International Drug Monitoring. *Drug Information Journal* 19:385–390.
Technology and the Regulation of Human Fertility (Special Issue)
  1987   *Technology in Society* 9:3–4.
Temin, Peter
  1980   *Taking Your Medicine: Drug Regulation in the United States.* Cambridge, Mass.: Harvard University Press.
Thapa, Shyam, David Hamill, and Philip Lampe
  1988   Continuation and Effectiveness of Program and Non-Program Methods of Family Planning in Rural Sri Lanka. Paper presented at the United Nations Expert Group Meeting on Methodologies for Measuring Contraceptive Use Dynamics, New York (December 5–7).
Tietze, Christopher, and Stanley K. Henshaw
  1986   *Induced Abortion: A World Review,* 6th ed. New York: Alan Guttmacher Institute.
Troen, Philip, Gabriel Bialy, and Kevin Catt
  1983   *Contraceptive Development: An Evaluation and Assessment of the State of the Science.* Washington, D.C.: U.S. Department of Health and Human Services, Institute for Child Health and Human Development.
Trussell, James, and Anne R. Pebley
  1984   The potential impact of changes in fertility on infant, child and maternal mortality. *Studies in Family Planning* 15(6):267–280.
Trussell, James, and Kathryn Kost
  1987   Contraceptive failure in the United States: A critical review of the literature. *Studies in Family Planning* 18(5):237–283.
Ulmann, A., and C. Dubois
  1986   Clinical trials with RU486. Editorial. *New England Journal of Medicine* (December 18).
United Nations
  1983   *Recent Levels and Trends in Contraceptive Use as Assessed in 1983.* New York: United Nations.
  1984   Recommendations for the Further Implementation of the World Population Plan of Action. UN Doc. E/Conf. 76.5. International Conference on Population, Mexico City.
  1987a World Contraceptive Use. Data chart prepared by the Population Division of the Department of International Economic and Social Affairs of the United Nations. United Nations, New York.

1987b   *Consolidated List of Products Whose Consumption and/or Sale Have Been Banned, Withdrawn, Severely Restricted or Not Approved by Governments* Second Issue, ST/ESA/192. New York: United Nations.

Urang, Sally
1983   The pill and its marketing offspring. *Chemical Business* (July 25):9–15.

U.S. Agency for International Development (AID)
1989   Users Guide to the Office of Population. Agency for International Development, Washington, D.C.

U.S. Congress
1983   FDA's Approval of the Today Contraceptive Sponge. Hearing before a Subcommittee of the Committee on Government Operations, House of Representatives, 98th Congress, First Session (July 13):130.
1987   H.R. 1115 (100th Congress, First Session).

U.S. Department of Commerce
1979   Model Uniform Product Liability Act. *Federal Register* 44(October 31):62717–62750.

U.S. Department of Health and Human Services
1980   Vaginal contraceptive drug products for over-the-counter human use: Establishment of a monograph; proposed rulemaking. *Federal Register* 45(241)(December 12):82014–82046.
1987   New drug, antibiotic, and biologic drug product regulations; final rule. *Federal Register* 52(March 19):8798–8847.

U.S. Department of Justice
1986   *Report of the Policy Working Group on the Causes, Extent and Policy Implications of the Current Crisis in Insurance Availability and Affordability.* (February). Washington D.C.: U.S. Government Printing Office.
1987   *An Update on the Liability Crisis and Tort Policy Working Group.* (March). Washington D.C.: U.S. Government Printing Office.

Van Keep, Pieter A., Kenneth Ellison Davis, and David de Wied
1987   *Contraception in the Year 2001.* New York: Excerpta Medica.

Vessey, M., M. Lawless, and D. Yeates
1982   Efficacy of different contraceptive methods. *Lancet* 1(8276):841–842.

Viel, Benjamin
1985   Induced Abortion in Latin America: Impact on Health. Symposium to honor Christopher Tietze, Berlin, Germany.

Wahren, Carl
1983   The role of industry, agencies and governments in research on fertility regulation: Past experience and future prospects. Pages 301–349 in E. Diczfalusy and A. Diczfalusy, eds., *Research on the Regulation of Human Fertility,* Volume 1. Copenhagen, Denmark: Scriptor.

Walsh, Sharon W.
1988   Liability bill losing momentum. *Washington Post* (Sunday, April 10).

Wardell, William M.
1979   The history of drug discovery development and regulation. In Robert I. Chien, ed., *Issues in Pharmaceutical Economics.* Lexington, Mass.: D.C. Heath and Company.

Watkins, Richard N.
  1986   Vaginal spermicides and congenital disorders: The validity of a study. *Journal of the American Medical Association* 256(22):3095.
Weisbord, Robert
  1975   *Genocide: Birth Control and the Black American.* Westport, Conn.: Greenwood Press and New York: The Two Continents Publishing Group.
Westoff, Charles F., Charles R. Hammerslough, and Lois Paul
  1987   Potential Impacts of Fertility and Abortion in Western Countries of Improvements in Contraception. Paper prepared for the European Population Conference, Jyvaskyla, Finland.
Westoff, Charles F., and Robert Parke
  1972   Aspects of Population Growth Policy. Commission on Population Growth and the American Future. Research Reports. Volume 6.
Westoff, Charles F., and Norman B. Ryder
  1977   *The Contraceptive Revolution.* Princeton, N.J.: Princeton University Press.
Westwood, Albert R.C., and Yukiko Sekine
  1988   Fostering creativity and innovation in an industrial R&D laboratory. *Research Technology Management* 31(4)(July–August):16–20.
Wiedhaup, Koenraad
  1988   View of Contraceptive Development. Background paper prepared for the Committee on Contraceptive Development, National Research Council and Institute of Medicine.
Wiggins, Steven N.
  1987   *The Cost of Developing a New Drug.* Washington, D.C.: Pharmaceutical Manufacturers Association.
William and Flora Hewlett Foundation
  1987   *Annual Report.* Menlo Park, Calif.
Winter, Ralph A.
  1988   The liability crisis and the dynamics of competitive insurance markets. *Yale Journal of Regulation* 5:455–499.
World Bank
  1984   *World Development Report 1984.* New York: Oxford University Press.
World Health Organization
  1982   World Health Organization Certification Scheme on the Quality of Pharmaceutical Products. World Health Organization PHARM/82.4, Geneva, Switzerland.
  1984   The Role of the Special Programme in the Drug Regulatory Process. Advisory Group Position Paper (September). Special Programme of Research, Development and Research Training in Human Reproduction.
  1985a   Facts about an implantable contraceptive: Memorandum from a World Health Organization meeting. *Bulletin of the World Health Organization* 63(3):485–494.
  1985b   Special Programme of Research, Development, and Research Training in Human Reproduction. 14th Annual Report (December).
  1986a   *Maternal Mortality Rates: A Tabulation of Available Information,* 2nd. ed. Geneva, Switzerland: World Health Organization.

1986b   Depot-Medroxy-Progesterone Acetate (DMPA) and cancer: Memorandum from a World Health Organization meeting. *Bulletin of the World Health Organization* 64(3):375–382.

1987   Special Programme of Research, Development and Research Training in Human Reproduction. (May). Proposed programme budget for the 1988–1989 biennium and estimates for 1990–1991.

1988   *Research in Human Reproduction: Biennial Report 1986–1987.*   Geneva, Switzerland: World Health Organization Special Programme of Research, Development and Research Training in Human Reproduction.

Zatuchni, Gerald I., Alfredo Goldsmith, and John J. Sciarra

1985   *Intrauterine Contraception: Advances and Future Prospects.*   Philadelphia, Penna.:   Harper & Row.

Legal Cases Related to Contraceptive Development

Baroldy v. Ortho Pharmaceutical Corp., 157 Ariz. 574, 760 P.2d 574 (1988)

Beyette v. Ortho Pharmaceutical Corp., 823 F.2d 990 (6th Cir. 1987)

Brochu v. Ortho Pharmaceutical Corp., 642 F.2d 652 (1st Cir. 1981)

Buck v. Bell, 274 U.S. 200 (1926)

Chambers v. G.D. Searle & Co., 441 F. Supp. 377 (D. Md. 1975), affirmed, 567 F.2d 269 (4th Cir. 1977)

Cobb v. Syntex Laboratories, Inc., 444 So. 2d 203 (La. App. 1983)

Collins v. Ortho Pharmaceutical Corp., 186 Cal. App. 3d 1194, 231 Cal. Rptr. 396 (5th Dist. 1986)

Dunkin v. Syntex Laboratories, Inc., 443 F. Supp. 121 (W.D. Tenn. 1977)

Eiser v. Feldman, 507 N.Y.S.2d 386 (App. Div. 1986)

Federal Insurance Co. v. Oak Industries, Sec. Law Rep. para. 92,519 (S.D.Cal. 1986)

Gillespie v. Thomasville Coca-Cola Bottling Co., 17 N.C. App. 545, 195 S.E.2d 45, cert. denied, 283 N.C. 393, 196 S.E.2d 275 (1973)

Goodson v. Searle Laboratories, 471 F. Supp. 546 (D. Conn. 1978)

Greenman v. Yuba Power Products, Inc., 59 Cal. 2d 57, 377 P.2d 897 (1963)

Griswold v. Connecticut, 431 U.S. 687 (1965)

Jackson Township, Muncipal Utilities Authority v. Hartford Accident and Indemnity Co., 186 N.J. Super. 156, 451 A.2d 990 (1982)

Jordan v. Ortho Pharmaceutical Corp., 696 S.W.2d 228 (Tex. App. 1985)

J.P.M. and B.M. v. Schmid Laboratories, Inc., 178 N.J. Super. 122, 428 A.2d 515 (1981)

175

Kociemba v. G.D. Searle & Co., No. 3-85-1599 (D. Minn. Sept. 13, 1988); 1988 U.S. Dist. LEXIS 10580

Lawson v. G.D. Searle & Co., 64 Ill. 2d 543, 356 N.E.2d 779 (1976)

Lukaszewicz v. Ortho Pharmaceutical Corp., 510 F. Supp. 961 (E.D. Wisc. 1981)

MacDonald v. Ortho Pharmaceutical Corp., 394 Mass. 131, 475 N.E.2d 65, cert. denied 106 S.Ct. 250 (1985)

McEwen v. Ortho Pharmaceutical Corp., 270 Ore. 375, 528 P.2d 522 (1974)

Marder v. G.D. Searle & Co., 630 F. Supp. 1087 (D. Md. 1986) aff'd sub nom.

May v. Parke Davis and Co., 142 Mich. App. 404, 370 N.W.2d 371 (1985)

Odgers v. Ortho Pharmaceutical Corp., 609 F. Supp. 867 (E.D. Mich. 1985)

Ortho Pharmaceutical Corp. v. Heath, 722 P.2d 410 (Colo. 1986)

Palmer v. A.H. Robins Co., Inc., 684 P.2d 187 (Colo. 1984)

Reeder v. Hammond, 125 Mich. App. 223, 336 N.W.2d 3 (1983)

Roe v. Wade, 410 U.S. 113 (1973)

Romero v. G.D. Searle & Co., 15 Prod. Safety & Liab. Rep. (BNA) 669 (Sept. 18, 1987), N.M. Dist. Ct., CV 84-02244 and CV 86-08903

Seley v. G.D. Searle & Co., 67 Ohio St. 2d 192, 423 N.E.2d 831 (1981)

Skinner v. Oklahoma, 316 U.S. 535 (1942)

Spinden v. Johnson & Johnson, 177 N.J. Super. 605, 427 A.2d 597 (1981)

Stephens v. G.D. Searle & Co., 602 F. Supp. 379 (E.D. Mich. 1985)

Taylor v. Wyeth Laboratories, Inc., 139 Mich. App. 389, 362 N.W.2d 293 (1984)

Vaughn v. G.D. Searle & Co., 272 Ore. 367, 536 P.2d 1247 (1975), cert. denied, 423 U.S. 1054 (1976)

Webster v. Reproductive Health Services, 109 S. Ct. 3040 (1989)

Wells v. Ortho Pharmaceutical Corp., 615 F. Supp. 262 (N.D. Ga. 1985), aff'd, 788 F.2d 741 (11th Cir. 1986), cert. denied, 93 L.Ed.2d 386 (1986)

Wheelahan v. G.D. Searle & Co., 814 F.2d 655 (4th Cir. 1987)

Wooderson v. Ortho Pharmaceutical Corp., 235 Kan. 387, 681 P.2d 1038, cert. denied, 469 U.S. 965 (1984)

Glossary

Beta blocking agent: drugs that prevent the release of adrenaline and therefore may cause bradycardia (slowing of the heart), decreased cardiac output, and lowered blood pressure.

Claims-made liability policy: policy that covers claims filed within the policy period for injuries that occurred during the policy period or within the retroactive period defined by the policy.

Clinical trial: a study of a drug or device (or drugs or devices) in human beings; it is usually intended to assess safety, effectiveness, route of administration, dosage, or other aspects of the drug or device.

Compensatory damages: such damages that compensate an injured party for the injury sustained.

Comprehensive general liability insurance: insurance that covers indemnity payments and legal expenses arising from a range of liabilities, including products liability.

Ectopic pregnancy: development of the fertilized ovum outside the uterine cavity.

Effective patent life: the length of time from the date of FDA approval until the date of patent expiration.

Endometrium: the mucous membrane lining the uterus.

Epididymis: the structure in the testes in which the spermatozoa are stored.

Estrogen: female sex hormone produced by the ovary and responsible for the development of female secondary sex characteristics; it also stimulates the growth of the endometrium during the menstrual cycle and is used to stop lactation and suppress ovulation.

177

Grandfather provisions: an exception to a restriction that allows all those already doing something to continue doing it, even if they would be stopped by the new restriction.

Investigational Device Exemption (IDE): an exemption that FDA issues permitting manufacturers of devices intended solely for investigational use to distribute these devices for such use on human subjects.

Investigational New Drug Application (IND): an application that a drug sponsor must submit to FDA before beginning tests of a new drug on humans. The IND contains the plan for the study as well as the drug's manufacturing information, structural formula, and animal test results. Compare New Drug Application.

Institutional review board (IRB): a committee of experts and lay persons at a hospital or research institution that, in the interest of protecting human subjects, reviews clinical research before it begins and as it progresses.

Insurance sublines: see Long-tailed lines of insurance.

In vitro fertilization: fertilization of an ovum outside the body in an artificial environment (such as a test tube).

Joint underwriting association (JUA): an incorporated association of insurance companies formed under statutory guidelines to provide a particular form of insurance to the public that is not readily available in the voluntary insurance market. All insurers operating in a state are required to participate as a condition of writing other coverages. JUA rates are regulated by state authorities. Deficits are usually funded by an assessment on participating insurers.

Learned intermediary rule: a common law rule under which a manufacturer of a prescription drug has discharged its duty to warn the consumer if it informs the medical profession, including both prescribing and treating physicians, of potential risks and contraindictions.

Long-tailed lines of insurance: lines of insurance for which several years may elapse between the alleged harmful act and the final disposition of all related claims, due to delay in the manifestation of the injury and in the disposition of the claims. Long-tailed liability claims may be separated from the circumstances that caused them by 25 years or more—e.g., diethylstilbestrol (DES)-related and asbestos-related claims.

Mutual insurance companies: insurance companies in which the policy holders have ownership and control.

New Chemical Entity (NCE): a pharmaceutical preparation that is the subject of a New Drug Application and whose active ingredient has not previously been the subject of such an application.

New Drug Application (NDA): an application requesting FDA approval to market a new drug for human use. The application consists principally of data from clinical trials and animal studies, which are evaluated from specific technical perspectives—chemistry, pharmacology, medical, statistics, and microbiology. Compare Investigational New Drug Application.

Occurrence liability policy: an insurance policy that covers claims no matter when they are filed, as long as the injury occurred during the period the policy was in effect.

Pelvic inflammatory disease (PID): ascending infection from the vagina or cervix to the uterus, fallopian tubes, and broad ligaments.

Preclinical trial: studies that test a drug in animals and other nonhuman test systems.

Premarketing approval (PMA): a private license granted to the applicant for marketing a particular medical device.

Products liability: legal responsibility of manufacturers and sellers to compensate buyers, users, and even bystanders for damages or injuries suffered because of defects in goods purchased.

Products liability insurance: liability coverage that protects manufacturers and suppliers from claims for accidents arising from the use of their products.

Professional liability insurance policy: insurance against claims for damages arising from professional activities of physicians, lawyers, accountants, and other professionals.

Progesterone: the hormone that prepares the uterus for the reception and development of the fertilized ovum.

Progestin: name used for certain synthetic or natural progesterones.

Prostaglandin: a group of naturally occurring, chemically related, long-chain hydroxy fatty acids that stimulate contractility of the uterine and other smooth muscles.

Proximate cause: the legally recognized cause of an injury or an event.

Pulmonary embolism: obstruction or occlusion of the pulmonary artery or one of its branches by a clot or foreign material derived from elsewhere in the body.

Punitive damages: damages awarded to injured party that are designed to punish a wrongdoer rather than simply compensate the injured party.

Reanastomosis: surgical operation to reverse tubal sterilization or vasectomy.

Restatement (Second) of Torts: a summary and explanation of major principles of contemporary tort law by the American Law Institute.

Risk retention groups: groups formed to pool and insure risk by setting aside their own money rather than buying insurance from an outside source.

Self-insurance: plan in which the insured sets aside sufficient sums to cover expected losses that may be sustained.

Sperm antigens: substances on or in the sperm that in certain circumstances elicit the production of antibodies.

Statutory law: body of law derived from legislative acts or statutes.

Strict liability: a concept in which a manufacturer or seller of a product is liable for any and all defective or hazardous conditions associated with the product that unduly threaten a consumer's personal safety, regardless of the care taken in product development and distribution.

Tail coverage: liability insurance that covers claims reported beyond the end of the policy period of a liability insurance policy written on a claims-made basis.

Testosterone: the hormone produced by the testes responsible for inducing and maintaining male secondary sex characteristics.

Third party coverage: insurance indemnifying the insured with respect to any loss that might be sustained as a result of his or her legal liability to others.

Tort law: law surrounding a private or civil wrong or injury, other than breach of contract, for which the court will provide a remedy in the form of an action for damages.

Toxicological testing: the testing of a substance in animals or other nonhuman test systems in order to assess its toxic or otherwise harmful effects.

Transdermal patches: patches impregnated with pharmaceutical agents that are placed on the skin as a system for sustained delivery of a medicament into the bloodstream.

Uniform Commercial Code: one of the uniform laws governing commercial transactions (e.g., sale of goods, commercial paper, investment securities).

Virucide: a chemical agent that neutralizes or destroys a virus.

Index